Gastroenterology in the Elderly

Guest Editors

NICHOLAS J. TALLEY, MD, PhD, FACP, FRACP, FRCP
ERIC G. TANGALOS, MD

GASTROENTEROLOGY CLINICS OF NORTH AMERICA

www.gastro.theclinics.com

September 2009 • Volume 38 • Number 3

SAUNDERS an imprint of ELSEVIER, Inc.

W.B. SAUNDERS COMPANY

A Division of Elsevier Inc.

Elsevier Inc. • 1600 John F. Kennedy Blvd., Suite 1800 • Philadelphia, Pennsylvania 19103-2899

http://www.theclinics.com

GASTROENTEROLOGY CLINICS OF NORTH AMERICA Volume 38, Number 3
September 2009 ISSN 0889-8553, ISBN-13: 978-1-4377-1219-3, ISBN-10: 1-4377-1219-3

Editor: Kerry Holland

Gastroenterology Clinics of North America (ISSN 0889-8553) is published quarterly by Elsevier Inc., 360 Park Avenue South, New York, NY 10010-1710. Months of issue are March, June, September, and December. Business and Editorial Offices: 1600 John F. Kennedy Blvd., Suite 1800, Philadelphia, PA 19103-2899. Customer Service Office: 6277 Sea Harbor Drive, Orlando, FL 32887-4800. Periodicals postage paid at New York, NY and additional mailing offices. Subscription prices are $256.00 per year (US individuals), $131.00 per year (US students), $385.00 per year (US institutions), $282.00 per year (Canadian individuals), $469.00 per year (Canadian institutions), $355.00 per year (international individuals), $181.00 per year (international students), and $469.00 per year (international institutions). Foreign air speed delivery is included in all *Clinics* subscription prices. All prices are subject to change without notice. **POSTMASTER**: Send address changes to *Gastroenterology Clinics of North America*, Elsevier Health Sciences Division, Subscription Customer Service, 3251 Riverport Lane, Maryland Heights, MO 63043. Telephone: 1-800-654-2452 (U.S. and Canada); 314-447-8871 (outside U.S. and Canada). Fax: 314-447-8029. E-mail: journalscustomerservice-usa@elsevier.com (for print support); journalsonlinesupport-usa@elsevier.com (for online support).

Reprints. For copies of 100 or more, of articles in this publication, please contact the Commercial Reprints Department, Elsevier Inc., 360 Part Avenue South, New York, New York 10010-1710. Tel. (212) 633-3813, Fax: (212) 462-1935, E-mail: reprints@elsevier.com.

Gastroenterology Clinics of North America is also published in Italian by Il Pensiero Scientifico Editore, Rome, Italy; and in Portuguese by Interlivros Edicoes Ltda., Rua Commandante Coelho 1085, 21250 Cordovil, Rio de Janeiro, Brazil.

Gastroenterology Clinics of North America is covered in *MEDLINE/PubMed (Index Medicus), Excerpta Medica, Current Contents/Clinical Medicine, Science Citation Index, ISI/BIOMED*, and *BIOSIS*.

Printed and bound by CPI Group (UK) Ltd, Croydon, CR0 4YY

Transferred to Digital Print 2011

Contributors

GUEST EDITORS

NICHOLAS J. TALLEY, MD, PhD, FACP, FRACP, FRCP
Chair, Department of Internal Medicine, and Consultant, Division of Gastroenterology and Hepatology, Mayo Clinic Florida, Jacksonville, Florida; and Professor of Medicine and Epidemiology, Mayo Clinic College of Medicine, Rochester, Minnesota

ERIC G. TANGALOS, MD
Consultant, Primary Care Internal Medicine, Mayo Clinic; and Professor of Medicine, Mayo Medical School, Rochester, Minnesota

AUTHORS

ERNEST P. BOURAS, MD
Assistant Professor, Mayo Clinic College of Medicine; Consultant, Division of Gastroenterology and Hepatology, Mayo Clinic, Jacksonville, Florida

JOHN R. CANGEMI, MD
Assistant Professor of Medicine, and Consultant, Division of Gastroenterology, Department of Medicine, Mayo Clinic Florida, Jacksonville, Florida

IAN McPHEE CHAPMAN, MBBS, FRACP, PhD
Associate Professor, Department of Medicine, University of Adelaide, Royal Adelaide Hospital, North Terrace, Adelaide, South Australia, Australia

IAN J. COOK, MBBS, MD(Syd), FRACP
Professor of Medicine, University of New South Wales; and Director, Department of Gastroenterology and Hepatology, St George Hospital, Kogarah, Sydney, New South Wales, Australia

ERIC J. DOZOIS, MD
Fellow, Division of Colon and Rectal Surgery, Mayo Clinic, Rochester, Minnesota

YAIR EDDEN, MD
Department of Colorectal Surgery, Cleveland Clinic, Weston, Florida

FELIX W. LEUNG, MD, FACG
Division of Gastroenterology, Department of Medicine, David Geffen School of Medicine at UCLA; and Sepulveda Ambulatory Care Center, Veterans Affairs Greater Los Angeles Healthcare System, North Hills, California

JOSEPH A. MURRAY, MD
Professor of Medicine and Immunology, Division of Gastroenterology and Hepatology, Department of Medicine, Mayo Clinic College of Medicine, Rochester, Minnesota

MICHAEL F. PICCO, MD, PhD
Consultant, Department of Medicine, Division of Gastroenterology, Mayo Clinic Florida, Jacksonville, Florida

SATISH S.C. RAO, MD, PhD, FRCP (LON)
Department of Internal Medicine, University of Iowa Carver College of Medicine, Iowa City, Iowa

SHADI RASHTAK, MD
Postdoctoral research fellow, Division of Gastroenterology and Hepatology, Department of Medicine, Mayo Clinic College of Medicine; and Department of Dermatology, Mayo Clinic College of Medicine, Rochester, Minnesota

LAWRENCE R. SCHILLER, MD
Digestive Health Associates of Texas; Program Director, Gastroenterology Fellowship, Baylor University Medical Center; and Clinical Professor, Department of Internal Medicine, University of Texas Southwestern Medical Center, Dallas, Texas

SHIRLEY S. SHIH, MD
Department of Colorectal Surgery, Cleveland Clinic, Weston, Florida

ERIC G. TANGALOS, MD
Consultant, Primary Care Internal Medicine, Mayo Clinic; and Professor of Medicine, Mayo Medical School, Rochester, Minnesota

JOHN G. TOUZIOS, MD
Associate Professor of Surgery, and Consultant, Division of Colon and Rectal Surgery, Mayo Clinic, Rochester, Minnesota

RENUKA VISVANATHAN, MBBS, FRACP, PhD
Associate Professor (Geriatric Medicine), Department of Medicine, University of Adelaide, The Queen Elizabeth Hospital Campus; Clinical Director, Aged & Extended Care Services, The Queen Elizabeth Hospital, Central Northern Adelaide Health Services, Woodville South, South Australia, Australia

STEVEN D. WEXNER, MD
Department of Colorectal Surgery, Cleveland Clinic, Weston, Florida

BARBARA J. ZAROWITZ, PharmD, FCCP, BCPS, CGP, FASCP
Professional Services, Omnicare, Inc., Livonia, College of Pharmacy and Health Sciences, Wayne State University, Detroit, Michigan

Contents

Minimizing frailty in older age is important to individuals and society, as the increasing prevalence of chronic disease is leading to greater disability and health care costs. Nutritional frailty can be defined as the disability that occurs in old age due to rapid, unintentional loss of body weight and sarcopenia (lack of lean mass). This article provides a brief overview of the prevalence and consequences of undernutrition, age-related changes to appetite, food intake, and body composition, the factors contributing to the development of anorexia and undernutrition, and recommended management strategies.

Although the aging process per se can produce measurable changes in the normal oropharyngeal swallow, these changes alone are rarely sufficient to cause clinically apparent dysphagia. The causes of oropharyngeal dysphagia in the elderly are predominantly neuromyogenic, with the most common cause being stroke. The evaluation of oropharyngeal dysphagia in the elderly involves early exclusion of structural abnormalities, detection of aspiration by videofluoroscopy which might dictate early introduction of nonoral feeding, and exclusion of underlying systemic and neuromyogenic causes that have specific therapies in their own right. Such conditions include Parkinson disease, myositis, myasthenia, and thyrotoxicosis. Management is best delivered by a multidisciplinary team involving physician, speech pathologist, nutritionist and, at times, a surgeon.

It has become apparent recently that celiac disease, once believed to be primarily a childhood disease, can affect people of any age. Epidemiologic studies have suggested that a substantial portion of patients are diagnosed after the age of 50. Indeed, in one study, the median age at the diagnosis was just under the age of 50 with one-third of new patients diagnosed being older than 65 years. The purpose of this review is to address the prevalence, clinical features, diagnosis, and consequences of celiac disease in the elderly. The authors also review management strategies for celiac disease and adjust these with emphasis on the particular nutritional and nonnutritional consequences or associations of celiac disease as they pertain to the elderly.

This article reviews the epidemiology, clinical manifestations, diagnosis, prognosis, and treatment of inflammatory bowel disease (IBD), which will grow in prevalence as the population ages. Prognosis of late-onset ulcerative colitis (UC) is generally similar to that of early-onset UC, whereas in Crohn disease it is probably better because of a tendency for colonic involvement. Disease complications are related more to the duration of the inflammatory bowel disease than the subject's current age. The diagnosis in elderly patients can be challenging due to the large number of conditions that mimic IBD on radiologic, endoscopic, and histologic testing. Distinguishing these conditions from IBD will significantly alter prognosis and treatment. Complications related to IBD and its treatment are common and must be recognized early to limit their impact in a vulnerable elderly population.

Chronic constipation is a common problem in the elderly, with a variety of causes, including pelvic floor dysfunction, medication effects, and numerous age-specific conditions. A stepwise diagnostic and therapeutic approach to patients with chronic constipation based on historical and physical examination features is recommended. Prudent use of fiber supplements and laxative agents may be helpful for many patients. Based on their capabilities, patients with pelvic floor dysfunction should be considered for pelvic floor rehabilitation (biofeedback), although efficacy in the elderly is uncertain. Clinical awareness and focused testing to identify the physiologic abnormalities underlying constipation, while being mindful of situations unique to the elderly, facilitate management, and improve patient outcomes.

Acute and chronic diarrheal disorders are common problems at all ages. It has been estimated that 5% to 7% of the population has an episode of acute diarrhea each year and that 3% to 5% have chronic diarrhea that lasts more than 4 weeks. It is likely that the prevalence of diarrhea is similar in older individuals. This article reviews the impact of diarrhea in the elderly, many of whom are less fit physiologically to withstand the effect of diarrhea on fluid balance and nutritional balance.

Fecal incontinence affects up to 20% of community-dwelling adults and more than 50% of nursing home residents, and is one of the major risk factors for elderly persons in the nursing home. Institutionalization itself is a risk factor (eg, immobility due to physical restraints). Management should focus on identifying and treating underlying causes, such as diet- or medication induced diarrhea, constipation, and fecal impaction. Use of absorbent pads and special undergarments is useful. Anorectal physiologic testing of nursing home residents has revealed an association between constipation, stool retention, and fecal incontinence. Impaired sphincter function (risk factor for fecal incontinence), decreased rectal sensation, and sphincter dyssynergia (risk factor for constipation and impaction) are found in a high proportion of incontinent nursing home residents. Biofeedback and sacral nerve stimulation may be useful in refractory patients and should be considered before colostomy in community-dwelling adults. Despite appropriate management, nursing home residents may remain incontinent because of dementia and health or restraint related immobility.

Colonic diverticulosis is a common, usually asymptomatic, entity of Western countries, with an incidence that increases with age. When these diverticula become infected and inflamed, patients can present with a wide variety of clinical manifestations. Management of acute, uncomplicated diverticulitis can often be treated successfully with antibiotics alone and the decision to proceed with more aggressive measures such as surgical intervention is made on a case-by-case basis. The treatment algorithm for diverticular disease continues to evolve as the pathophysiology, etiology, and natural history of the disease becomes better understood.

Mesenteric ischemia in the elderly is an uncommon but often fatal disorder for which the prognosis depends entirely on the speed and accuracy of the diagnosis. A high index of suspicion is required as the early signs and symptoms, at a time when ischemic changes are reversible, are typically nonspecific or absent. This article reviews the clinical spectrum of mesenteric ischemia in the elderly with particular emphasis on the varied presentations, evaluation, and management of ischemic disorders of the intestines.

Colonic ulcerations can affect the entire colon and rectum, and have variable clinical presentation according to the anatomic location and underlying pathology. Diverse causes may lead to colonic ulceration, such as inflammatory bowel diseases, oral drugs (mostly nonsteroidal anti-inflammatory drugs), local or diffuse ischemia, and different intestinal microorganisms. An ulcer may also herald a concealed malignant disease. In most cases, colonic ulcerate is associated with diffuse colitis in the acute setup or with inflammatory bowel diseases, and to the lesser extent the ulceration is defined as solitary. This article focuses on two of the less commonly diagnosed diseases: solitary rectal ulcer syndrome and stercoral ulceration, both related to local tissue ischemia and often seen in the elderly population.

Gastrointestinal (GI) manifestations in older adults can be caused or alleviated by drug therapy. GI medications, such as proton pump inhibitors and histamine-2 receptor antagonists, are among the most commonly used medications in long-term care facilities in the United States. This article reviews the alterations in pharmacokinetic disposition of medications that occur with aging and highlights the pharmacology of commonly used GI drugs. Selected GI conditions that are drug induced and preventable are identified, and recommendations for GI drugs to be avoided in older adults are provided.

THE CLINICS ARE NOW AVAILABLE ONLINE!

Access your subscription at:
www.theclinics.com

ISSUES OF RELATED INTEREST

Clinics in Geriatric Medicine, November 2007 (Volume 23, Issue 4)
Gastroenterology
T.S. Dharmarajan, Guest Editor

Preface

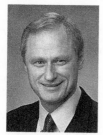 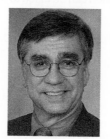

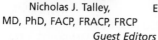

Nicholas J. Talley,
MD, PhD, FACP, FRACP, FRCP

Eric G.Tangalos, MD

Guest Editors

This issue of the *Gastroenterology Clinics of North America* devoted to gastroenterology in the elderly is timely and important, because the evidence is overwhelming: the demographics of the population in the United States and worldwide are rapidly changing, with a growing proportion of older people. With this change will come an accentuation of many clinical disease states. Baby boomers have just started to retire; by the year 2030, there will be 27 million people aged 65 years and older in the United States. Their maladies, along with their desire to stay young and healthy, create a tension that only intensifies with each passing year, and gastroenterologists will need to be able to expertly tackle their relevant medical issues.

We have brought together experts in gastroenterology and gastrointestinal surgery, who cover 11 key topics. We tasked authors to share with us their understanding of the clinical illnesses that confront the aging gut. In every article, emerging evidence that is unique to a geriatric population has been included where possible. In many instances, we have found that such data are still not robust and urge that efforts with regard to research and aging be ongoing.

We have tried to balance the science of aging with what is known about clinical geriatrics and gastroenterology. The elderly carry a burden of comorbid disease that adds complexity to every interaction and intervention. Our authors help address the science and art of caring for this unique population.

With some conditions as the population ages, there is a higher incidence and prevalence of disease, such as constipation and colon cancer. In other situations, we must be ever more vigilant so as not to miss problems, such as "late onset" celiac disease. *Clostridium difficile* and other infections are now more commonplace in the elderly and will likely be an even bigger problem with continuing antibiotic use and institutionalization. One can only imagine what a similar text might look like in another 10 or 20 years.

We hope you will agree that this issue offers the most current information available regarding important disease states and clinical practice in geriatric gastroenterology. It should serve as an appropriate reference for primary care providers and subspecialists

Gastroenterol Clin N Am 38 (2009) xi–xii
doi:10.1016/j.gtc.2009.07.001
0889-8553/09/$ – see front matter © 2009 Elsevier Inc. All rights reserved.

alike. Our authors have taken the time to provide plenty of detail but have avoided becoming bogged down in some of the finer points that have less practical value. We hope you will find that the information can be taken to the bedside and immediately applied.

Nicholas J. Talley, MD, PhD, FACP, FRACP, FRCP
Department of Internal Medicine
Mayo Clinic Florida
4500 San Pablo Road
Jacksonville, FL 32224, USA

Eric G. Tangalos, MD
Department of Medicine, Primary Care Internal Medicine
Mayo Clinic
200 First Street SW Rochester
MN 55905, USA

E-mail addresses:
talley.nicholas@mayo.edu (N.J. Talley)
tangalos@mayo.edu (E.G. Tangalos)

Undernutrition and Anorexia in the Older Person

Renuka Visvanathan, MBBS, FRACP, PhD[a,b],
Ian McPhee Chapman, MBBS, FRACP, PhD[a,*]

KEYWORDS

• Anorexia • Undernutrition • Sarcopenia • Obesity • Elderly

As populations age, health policies and research agendas are focusing increasingly on healthy aging. Minimizing frailty in older age is important to individuals and society, as the increasing prevalence of chronic disease is leading to greater disability and health care costs. Widely used frailty scores, such as the Fried Frailty Score and the Rockwood Frailty Index, include weight loss among their parameters, which indicates the importance of healthy nutrition in the attainment of healthy aging.[1,2] In keeping with this notion, a recent study found that low nutrient intake was independently associated with frailty.[3] Nutritional frailty can be defined as the disability that occurs in old age due to rapid, unintentional loss of body weight and sarcopenia (lack of lean mass).[1] A better understanding of the pathophysiology of undernutrition in older people is necessary to aid the development of effective prevention and intervention strategies, and achievement of healthy aging. This article provides a brief overview of the prevalence and consequences of undernutrition, age-related changes to appetite, food intake, and body composition, factors contributing to the development of anorexia and undernutrition, and recommended management strategies. Although malnutrition includes obesity, this topic is only briefly discussed in the context of older people in this article.

Funding support: Supported by project grants to A/Prof. Visvanathan of the Vincent Fairfax Family Foundation (through the Royal Australasian College of Physicians), the Bernie Lewis Foundation (through the Queen Elizabeth Hospital Research Foundation), and the University of Adelaide, Faculty of Health Science.
Supported by a project grant from the National Health and Medical Research Council of Australia to A/Prof. Chapman.
[a] Department of Medicine, University of Adelaide, Level 6 Eleanor Harrold Building, Royal Adelaide Hospital, North Terrace, Adelaide, South Australia 5000, Australia
[b] Aged and Extended Care Services, Central Northern Adelaide Health Services, Level 8B, The Queen Elizabeth Hospital, Woodville Road, Woodville South, South Australia 5011, Australia
* Corresponding author.
E-mail address: ian.chapman@adelaide.edu.au (I. McPhee Chapman).

PREVALENCE OF UNDERNUTRITION

Prevalence figures for undernutrition among older people quoted in the literature vary depending on the assessment method used. There are multiple ways of assessing nutrition and undernutrition in older people, none of them universally accepted. To enable comparisons across different settings, prevalence figures quoted here are nutritional risk as assessed by the widely used Mini Nutritional Assessment (MNA; discussed later). The reported prevalence of nutritional risk in older people is approximately 45% in the community, 45% to 51% in domiciliary care settings, 50% to 82% in hospitals, and between 84% and 100% in residential care facilities.[4–9] There is clearly a relationship between increasing frailty and increasing nutritional risk.

ADVERSE CONSEQUENCES OF UNDERNUTRITION

Undernutrition in older people is associated with multiple adverse health consequences, including impaired muscle function, decreased bone mass, immune dysfunction, anemia, reduced cognitive function, poor wound healing, delayed recovery from surgery, and ultimately, increased mortality.[10] In the SENECA (Survey in Europe on Nutrition and the Elderly, a Concerted Action) study, subjects with better MNA scores (MNA $\geq$24) had significantly lower mortality (odds ratio: 0.35, 95% CI: 0.18–0.66) than subjects at nutritional risk (MNA <24).[11] Older people often perceive entry into residential care as a bad outcome; individuals are at significant risk of this following an acute illness. Acute illness (inflammation) and prolonged bed rest results in increased protein catabolism, muscle loss, and loss of physical function. In one study of 908 community-dwelling elderly hospitalized patients, elderly malnourished subjects were 3 times more likely than nourished subjects to be subsequently institutionalized (20.3% MNA <17 versus 7.7% MNA $\geq$24; $P<.001$).[12] A study by the authors' group also confirmed that undernourished (MNA <24) community-dwelling older people in receipt of domiciliary care services were more likely to be hospitalized and spend longer in hospital than their nourished counterparts.[9] Individuals experiencing poor nutritional health are clearly at a higher risk of adverse health outcomes, increased frailty, and reduced quality of life.

RECOGNIZING UNDERNUTRITION

There is no generally accepted gold standard method for the diagnosis of undernutrition in older people. The MNA, the Malnutrition Universal Screening Tool, and the Subjective Global Assessment are commonly used screening tools.[13–15] Common to most screening tools are questions about weight loss and the body mass index (BMI), calculated as the weight in kilograms divided by height in meters squared. Appetite reduction usually precedes weight loss. The Simplified Nutritional Appetite Questionnaire comprises four questions on appetite, timing of eating, and frequency of meals and taste, and has a high sensitivity and specificity (both >75%) in predicting future 5% weight loss in older people.[16] The use of this tool in otherwise healthy older people can identify those who require assessment to prevent weight loss. Screening should be followed by a more in-depth assessment by experienced clinicians to confirm the diagnosis. A detailed assessment usually involves a combination of the following: anthropometric measures, questions regarding weight loss, food intake assessment, medication history, and measurement of blood parameters such as serum albumin, hematocrit, lymphocyte count, total cholesterol, and serum folate (all of which tend to be reduced in malnutrition).[17] Although there is ongoing debate about the best screening tool to use, a greater challenge is to be aware of undernutrition in older people, so that the diagnosis is considered, some screening is undertaken, and assessment and intervention follow.

Weight Loss and Body Mass Index

On average, body weight and hence BMI increase through adult life until about age 50 to 60 years, after which they decline.[18] One explanation for the decline in body weight after the age of 50 to 60 years detected in cross-sectional studies is the premature demise of obese individuals. This finding is a factor, but even in longitudinal studies there is evidence of a decrease in body weight from the age of 60 years onwards. In one prospective study of community-dwelling Americans, men aged 65 years and older lost on average 0.5% of their body weight per year and 13.1% of the group had weight loss of 4% or more per year.[19] Because of this weight loss and the premature death of obese individuals, the prevalence of overweight and obesity declines after about age 65 years, whereas the prevalence of underweight increases. For instance in the 1997 to 1998 US National Health Interview Survey of 68,556 adults, more people aged 75 years and older than those 45 to 64 years old were "underweight" (BMI <18.5 kg/m^2; 5 versus 1.6%) and substantially fewer were "overweight" (BMI >25 kg/m^2; 61.1 versus 47.2%).[20]

Clinicians must look out for weight loss in older people, as it occurs commonly, and whether unintentional or intentional (probable) weight loss is associated with poor outcomes (see Omran and Morley[21] for review). For example, the Cardiovascular Health Study in the United States prospectively evaluated 4714 home-dwelling subjects without cancer aged 65 years and older.[1] By 3 years, 17% of the subjects had lost 5% or more of their initial body weight. During the next 4 years this group had significantly greater total (2.09× ↑ [95% CI 1.67–2.62]) and risk-adjusted mortality (1.67× ↑ [1.29–2.15]) than the stable weight group. This increased risk occurred irrespective of the starting weight and apparently irrespective of whether weight was lost intentionally or not. Similar results were seen in the Systolic Hypertension in the Elderly Program (SHEP) study, in which subjects who lost 1.6 kg/y or more had a 4.9 times greater death rate (95% CI 3.5–6.8) than those without significant weight change. The association between increased mortality and weight loss was present even in the subjects who were heaviest at baseline (BMI ≥31) and was independent of baseline weight. Subjects with a low baseline weight (BMI < 23.6 kg/m^2) who lost more than 1.6 kg/y had a mortality rate of 22.6%, almost 20 times greater than the mortality rate of those with a baseline BMI of 23.6 to 28 kg/m^2 whose weight remained stable. Therefore, weight loss in an older person of initially low body weight is associated with a particularly bad outcome. This situation perhaps occurs because such weight loss is occurring in individuals who are already sarcopenic or because this weight loss is a reflection of underlying disease or inflammation, and therefore more likely to be unintentional. The tendency for older people to lose weight is variable, with lean individuals probably most at risk.[22] In keeping with this tendency, underweight older individuals irrespective of current weight stability should be comprehensively evaluated to minimize factors that may contribute to weight loss and poor nutritional health.

It is uncertain whether *intentional* weight loss really does result in adverse health outcomes in older people. There are epidemiologic studies to suggest this. The issue is especially important when advising older, overweight people about whether they should attempt to lose weight. Obesity is now a common health condition in older people and is increasing in prevalence. Obesity in older people is associated with increased disability, particularly from lower limb arthritis. In the English Longitudinal Study of Ageing (ELSA), 3793 individuals aged 65 years and older had BMI measured and were followed for a mean of 5 years 1 month.[23] In this study, obese men and women had increased relative risks of reporting difficulties with their activities of daily living (men: relative risk [RR] 1.99, 95% CI 1.42–2.78; women: RR 1.66, 95% CI 1.25–2.19) and having impaired physical function (men: RR 1.51, 95% CI 1.05–2.16; women: RR 1.51, 95% CI 1.14–2.00) in comparison to individuals with BMI between 20 and 24.9 kg/m^2 (reference group). This risk increased between 1.5 and 2 times in severely obese (BMI ≥35 kg/m^2) individuals. There is evidence that weight loss in overweight older people is associated with improved quality of life. In the Nurses Health Study weight loss in initially overweight women was associated with improved physical function and vitality as well as decreased bodily pain.[24] Therefore older, overweight people will often, appropriately, want to lose weight. When weight is lost, however, there is a propensity to lose lean tissue as well as fat. The loss of this lean tissue, mainly muscle and bone, has several adverse effects in older people.[25] Even when weight is regained, the gain in lean mass does not make up for the loss during the weight-loss period.[25] Therefore, advice to older people to lose weight should be given cautiously and only to achieve a specific goal (eg, better mobility). Ideally the weight loss should be achieved in a way that preserves lean tissue as much as possible, by including an exercise component and optimizing bone protection with adequate calcium and vitamin D intake. Villareal et al have shown that weight can be lost with preservation of muscle mass in obese, older people, with a 6-month program of behavioral therapy in conjunction with exercise training three times per week.[26]

The evidence that deliberate weight loss by overweight, older people prolongs their lives is weaker. For example, in the ELSA study individuals with BMI between 30 and 35 kg/m^2 did not have increased mortality risk compared with the reference group. An increase in mortality risk was only seen for men with morbid obesity (BMI ≥35 kg/m^2). Even after excluding from that study individuals with large weight loss (5% or greater), with baseline disability, who smoked, with poor or fair baseline health, and with one or more comorbidities at baseline, there was no association between mortality and weight except in the most obese. This lack of association in older people has been reported in many other studies.[27] In terms of mortality and obese older individuals, the findings in various studies have been variable with a recent systematic review concluding that there is only a modest (about 10%) increase in mortality risk.[27] In the setting of chronic disease, obese individuals have a better prognosis than those with the ideal weight and this phenomenon has been described as the "obesity paradox."[28] It may be that those individuals with chronic disease and a higher BMI are protected by having less inflammation and more lean mass. Perhaps obese individuals seek treatment sooner and therefore have better prognosis. There may also be a selection bias in that more susceptible obese individuals may have died before study enrollment, and those remaining to participate in studies are more robust and have some sort of protective factors.

The distribution of adipose tissue is believed to be more important than the actual amount of fat tissue, and it is therefore not surprising that there are conflicting results in relation to mortality when the less accurate surrogate measure of BMI is used. The BMI or body weight does not allow clinicians to account for the relative amounts and differing effects of lean and fat mass. In the British Regional Heart Study, 4107 men (age 60–79 years) were reexamined in their 20th year of follow-up.[29] Mean follow-up from the time of reexamination was 6 years with a total of 713 deaths during this time. Men with underweight BMI (<18.5 kg/m^2) had the highest mortality but those who were overweight or obese had no increased risk of mortality in comparison to the ideal weight (18.5–24.9 kg/m^2) group after adjusting for indicators of ill health predictive of mortality. In this study, even after adjusting for BMI and mid arm circumference (MAC) there was, however, a strong positive association seen between increasing waist circumference (WC) and mortality (WC >102 cm; RR 1.53, 95% CI 1.15–2.05). In this study the association between WC and waist to hip ratio and mortality risk became significant only following adjustment for lean mass as measured by MAC. Clearly a lack of muscle mass and increased abdominal adiposity is associated with increased mortality risk in older men. Those with the lowest mortality risk were those with low WC (≤102 cm) and medium (24.92–26.42 cm) to high (>26.42 cm) MAC. Individuals with low MAC irrespective of WC had increased mortality risk. Increased mortality risk was also seen in individuals with medium and high MAC and increased WC.

PATHOPHYSIOLOGY OF UNDERNUTRITION

In general the reasons for undernutrition in older people are multiple and can broadly be categorized into age-related impairments of homeostasis, nonphysiologic causes, and physiologic causes such as sarcopenia and anorexia. These are discussed in subsequent sections.

Age-Related Impairment of Homeostasis

Healthy aging is associated with a physiologic decline in energy (food) intake and a reduction in function of homeostatic mechanisms that work in younger people to restore food intake in response to anorectic insults. As an illustration, Roberts and colleagues[30] underfed young and old men by 3.17 MJ/d (≈750 kcal/d) for 21 days and this was accompanied by weight loss in the young and old. After the underfeeding period the men were allowed to again eat ad libitum. The young men ate more than at baseline (before underfeeding) and quickly returned to normal weight, whereas the old men did not compensate, returned only to their baseline intake, and did not regain the weight they had lost. The combination of age-related physiologic anorexia and impaired homeostasis means older people do not respond as well as young adults to acute undernutrition. In consequence, after an anorectic insult (for example, major surgery), older people are likely to take longer than young adults to regain the lost weight, remain undernourished longer, and be more susceptible to subsequent superimposed illnesses, such as infections. Without aggressive intervention, there is a predisposition to a spiral of decline toward increasing frailty.

Nonphysiologic Factors

Similar to other geriatric syndromes (ie, falls), there are numerous intrinsic and extrinsic nonphysiologic factors contributing to poor nutritional health in older people (**Box 1**).[31,32] These factors are frequently overlooked when attempting to manage undernutrition in older people, and this may be a major reason for treatment failure.

Sarcopenia

With increasing age there is loss of skeletal muscle mass, quality, and strength. Muscle cross-sectional area decreases by approximately 40% between the ages of 20 and 60 years[33] and muscle strength is 20% to 40% lower in healthy men and women in their seventh and eighth decades than in their young adult counterparts.[33] Not only are there altered central and peripheral nervous system innervations but also influences from other factors such as decreased physical activity, altered hormonal status, inflammation, and decreased caloric and protein intake.[33] Inflammatory cytokines such as interleukin (IL)-6 are implicated in muscle mass loss (sarcopenia or cachexia), strength loss, and the development of disability.[34] Tumor necrosis factor-α (TNF-α) and IL-1β stimulate the release of IL-6.[34] One could also argue that reduced

Box 1
Nonphysiologic factors contributing to undernutrition in older people

Intrinsic factors

    Oral health

        Mouth ulcers

        Oral candida

        Poor dentition

    Gastrointestinal

        Esophagitis

        Esophageal stricture

        Achalasia

        Peptic ulcer disease/atrophic gastritis

        Constipation

        Colitis

        Malabsorption

    Neurologic

        Dementia

        Parkinson disease

        Cerebrovascular disease

    Psychological

        Alcoholism

        Bereavement

        Depression

        Cholesterol phobia

    Endocrinology

        Thyrotoxicosis

        Hypothyroidism

        Hypoadrenalism

        Hyperparathyroidism

    Other medical (cachexia)

        Cardiac failure, chronic obstructive airways disease, renal failure

        Inflammatory athropathies

        Infection: HIV, malignancy

Extrinsic factors

    Social factors

        Poverty

        Lack of transport

        Inability to shop

        Inability to prepare and cook meals

        Inability to feed

Social isolation

Lack of social support

Failure to cater to ethnic/food preferences

Medications (this list is not exhaustive)

Nausea/vomiting: antibiotics, opiates, digoxin, theophylline, nonsteroidal anti-inflammatory drugs (NSAIDs)

Anorexia: antibiotics, digoxin

Hypogeusia: metronidazole, calcium channel blockers, angiotensin-converting enzyme inhibitors, metformin

Early satiety: anticholinergic drugs, sympathomimetic agents

Reduced feeding ability: sedatives, opiates, psychotropic agents

Dysphagia: potassium supplements, NSAIDs, biphosphonates, prednisolone

Constipation: opiates, iron supplements, diuretics

Diarrhea: laxatives, antibiotics

Hypermetabolism: thyroxin, ephedrine

Data from Chapman IM. Endocrinology of anorexia of ageing. Best Pract Res Clin Endocrinol Metab 2004;18:437–52. MacIntosh C, Morley JE, Chapman IM. The anorexia of aging. Nutrition 2000;16:983–5.

caloric and protein intake may in part be driven by the anorexia of aging, which is described subsequently. There have been informative reviews on this topic.[33,35]

The progressive loss of skeletal muscle mass with increasing age, which can be up to 3 kg of lean body mass per decade after age 50 years, is accompanied by a progressive increase in fat tissue. Normal aging is associated with an increase in fat mass that peaks at approximately age 65 years in men and later in women.[36] Therefore, on average, older people at any given weight have substantially more body fat than young adults, indeed approximately twice as much in 75-year-old men as in 20-year-old men of the same weight.[36] Body fat is also distributed differently in older adults. A greater proportion of body fat in older than younger people is intrahepatic, intramuscular, and intra-abdominal versus subcutaneous,[37] changes that in younger people are associated with increased insulin resistance and adverse metabolic outcomes.[38] Given the increasing prevalence of obesity in middle-aged individuals, more people are entering old age with body fat stores already high. Coupled with the age-related loss of lean tissue, this means that sarcopenia and obesity (sarcopenic obesity) commonly coexist in older people. Sarcopenic obesity seems to be associated with worse health outcomes than sarcopenia or obesity alone.[39] Current definitions of sarcopenic obesity are based on the amount of lean mass and fat mass in an individual, derived from body composition measurements. These measures, although useful, do not account for differences in the quality of the muscle tissue, muscle strength, and the distribution of the fat tissue. Assessment of these criteria may further enhance the prognostic significance or these measures.[36]

The Physiologic Anorexia of Aging

Appetite loss

The "anorexia of aging" is a term used to refer to the physiologic reduction in appetite and food intake that accompanies normal aging.[1] The appetite loss and reduced oral intake seen with increasing age often predates the development of weight loss and undernutrition.[21] In comparison with younger people, healthy older people are less hungry and more full before meals, consume smaller and more monotonous meals more slowly, eat fewer snacks between meals, and become more rapidly satiated after eating a standard meal.[22,40] Average daily energy intake has been reported to decrease by up to 30% between 20 and 80 years.[21] For example, a decline in energy intake of 1321 calories/d in men and 629 calories/d in women between the ages and 20 and 80 years was reported in the 1989 cross-sectional American National Health and Nutrition Examination Survey, NHANES III.[41] Much of the age-related decrease in energy is probably a response to the decline in energy expenditure that also occurs as people get older. In many individuals, however, the decrease in energy intake is greater than the decrease in energy expenditure, so body weight is lost.

Alteration to taste and smell

Taste and smell are important in making eating pleasurable. In animals, aging is associated with altered function of ion channels, and receptors result that mediate taste and changes to taste cell membranes.[42] The sense of taste probably declines with age in humans but the results of studies are variable.[43] The number of fibers in the olfactory bulb and the number of olfactory receptors decrease with age.[44] With aging, increased receptor cell death is noted, whereas regeneration of olfactory receptor neurons is reduced.[45] In consequence, after the age of 50 years the sense of smell deteriorates in humans. In one study, compared with only 10% of subjects younger than 50 years of age, more than 60% of subjects aged 65 to 80 years and more than 80% of subjects aged 80 years or older had major reductions in their sense of smell.[44] The decline in sense of smell decreases food intake in the elderly and influences the type of food eaten, most likely resulting in a reduced interest in intake of food and a less varied, more monotonous diet. Sensory-specific satiety is the normal decline in pleasantness of the taste of a particular food after it has been consumed, resulting in a shift to other food choices during a meal and promoting the intake of a more varied, nutritionally balanced diet. The capacity to develop sensory-specific satiety is reduced in older people, perhaps due to reduced taste and smell, and this may contribute to a less varied diet and reduced energy intake in older people.[46]

Gut mechanisms

Aging is associated with cell loss in the myenteric plexus of the human esophagus and a decline in conduction velocity within visceral neurons.[43] The consequent reduction in sensory perception may contribute to reduced food intake by inhibiting the positive stimuli for feeding. The elderly frequently complain of increased fullness and early satiation during a meal. This complaint may also be related to changes in gastrointestinal sensory function; aging is associated with reduced sensitivity to gastrointestinal tract distension. If anything, reduced sensitivity to the satiating effects of distension might be expected to increase, not decrease, food intake in older people. Nevertheless, proximal gastric distension has been found to have similar effects on food intake in healthy older and young adults. Therefore the role, if any, of impairment of gastric sensory function in causing the anorexia of aging is unknown.

Aging is associated with a slowing of gastric emptying, which may relate to altered activity of nitric oxide (NO) and hence with the development of anorexia.[43] Altered fundic NO results in an impaired gastric accommodation response. Peripheral NO causes receptive and adaptive relaxation of the stomach, leading to dilation of the fundus and ultimately slower gastric emptying. Clarkston and colleagues[47] found that healthy older subjects were less hungry and more satiated after a meal than young subjects, and that postprandial hunger was inversely related to the rate of gastric emptying. When small meals are consumed, as is the case with most older people, the gastric emptying rate between young and old is not different.[43] Delayed gastric emptying in older people, which is usually seen when meals with large energy content is consumed may, in part, result from enhanced release of small intestinal hormones such as cholecystokinin (CCK) (discussed later).

Gut transit time is not affected in healthy older people. Healthy older people do have slower phase III migration velocities and more frequent "propagated contractions" in the small intestine, but no differences in duration of postprandial motility or amplitude or frequency of fasting or postprandial pressure waves.

Neuroendocrine mechanisms

Appetite and food intake (**Table 1**) are heavily influenced by actions of components of the neuroendocrine axis, including the opioids, noradrenaline, neuropeptide Y, the orexins, galanin, and ghrelin, and the inhibitory effect of corticotrophin-releasing factor, serotonin, CCK, and possibly insulin. A more detailed review is available elsewhere.[43]

Central

Opioids There is evidence that aging is associated with a reduced opioid feeding drive.[48] Elderly patients with idiopathic, senile anorexia have lower plasma and cerebrospinal fluid (CSF) β-endorphin concentrations than normal weight, aged-matched controls.[49]

Neuropeptide Y Neuropeptide Y (NPY) is synthesized in the peripheral nervous system and brain, and strongly stimulates food intake. CSF NPY levels increase with healthy aging in women, and plasma and CSF levels are increased in elderly people with idiopathic anorexia.[49]

Galanin Galanin is a peptide hormone located in the brain and periphery that stimulates food intake. Declining galanin levels are unlikely to contribute to the anorexia of aging,[50] but reduced sensitivity to galanin might.

Orexins (hypocretins) Orexin A and B (hypocretin-1 and -2) are neuropeptides synthesized in the hypothalamus and are involved with feeding and sleep. Plasma orexin concentrations apparently increase, not decrease, with age in healthy humans,[51] although the effect of age on brain and receptor levels and the sensitivity to orexin is not known. Orexin deficiency causes narcolepsy in animals and humans, and hypophagia and weight loss in animals,[51] whereas orexin increases food intake.[52]

Cocaine-amphetamine–regulated transcript Cocaine-amphetamine–regulated transcript (CART) is a peptide widely distributed through the brain including the hypothalamus In animals central CART administration reduces feeding and blocks NPY-induced feeding. The effect of aging on CART in humans is unknown.

Peripheral hormones, including gut peptides

Cholecystokinin CCK is present in the hypothalamus, cortex, and midbrain, and is released from the lumen of the intestine in response to nutrients in the gut particularly fat and protein.[43] The administration of doses producing plasma CCK concentrations within the physiologic range results in suppression of food intake, whereas the administration of CCK antagonists increases food intake in animals and young, adult humans.[53] CCK also slows gastric emptying. The satiating effects of CCK seem to

Table 1
Factors contributing to the anorexia of aging

Factors	Effects
Nonhormonal factors	
Diminished sense of smell and taste	Decreased oral intake
Reduced sensory-specific satiety	More monotonous diet
Increased cytokine activity	Reduced food intake, cachexia
Alteration in gastrointestinal function	Delayed gastric emptying, altered gastric distribution of food
Hormonal factors	
Opioid: decreased opioid activity, not proven in humans	Exogenous opioid increases food intake in adult humans
Testosterone: decrease with age	Stimulates increase in muscle mass. Unclear if this results in functional gains
Ghrelin: possible decrease with age, not proven in humans	Stimulates food intake, gastric emptying, and growth hormone release.[81,82] Worsens glucose metabolism in humans[83]
Neuropeptide Y: possible decrease with aging, little evidence in humans	Has not been administered in humans. Increases food intake in animals
Cocaine-amphetamine–related transcript: changes in human not proven	In animals central administration reduces feeding
Cholecystokinin: satiating effects seem to increase with age	Exogenous administration reduces food intake in animals and humans
Leptin: levels increase with aging but may be mostly explained by increase adiposity and reduced testosterone levels	Administration suppresses food intake and appetite
Peptide YY: effect of age on Peptide YY is unclear	Administration reduces food intake and weight in human. Not a consistent finding

Data from Chapman IM. The anorexia of aging. Clin Geriatr Med 2007;23:735.

increase with age and in most studies plasma CCK concentrations are higher in healthy older than young adults.[54] In comparison to healthy age-matched controls, elderly people with idiopathic anorexia have significantly higher plasma levels and nonsignificantly higher CSF levels of CCK.[49] In one study, intravenous administration of CCK-8 acutely suppressed food intake twice as much (31% versus 15%, $P = .02$) in older versus young adult healthy, human subjects.[54] The possible use of CCK antagonists to increase energy intake in undernourished older people is supported by these findings.

Glucagon-like peptide 1 Glucagon-like peptide 1 (GLP-1) is released by the lining of the intestine in response to nutrient ingestion, particularly carbohydrates, and it slows gastric emptying.[43] GLP-1 stimulates insulin secretion and, together with gastric inhibitory peptide, is one of the incretin hormones. Administration of GLP-1 to humans increases feelings of fullness and reduces food intake.[55] The effects of aging on plasma GLP-1 concentrations[56] and the effects of aging on the satiating effects of GLP-1 are unknown.

Peptide YY Peptide YY (PYY) is a peptide hormone present in the brain and is released from the bowel in response to fat and carbohydrate in the small intestine. Intravenous infusion of PYY to normal weight and obese humans younger than 50 years of age, in doses that produce postprandial blood levels, reduced short-term food intake by approximately 30% in one study, although these results have not been easily reproducible.[57] Therefore although identified as a potential contributor to the development of the anorexia of aging, this result is not confirmed.[43]

Leptin Leptin is produced predominantly in adipose tissue and circulates in amounts directly related to the size of fat stores. Leptin administration to obese people has resulted in only minor weight loss and most likely this is due to leptin resistance.[43] Plasma leptin concentrations in humans often increase with aging and to a large extent this is due to the increased fat mass that accompanies aging.[58] Leptin levels may also be increased as a result of decreases in circulating testosterone concentrations in men. Plasma leptin levels are inversely related to plasma testosterone; testosterone therapy reduces, and inhibition of testosterone production increases, circulating leptin levels.[59] Aging may be accompanied by leptin resistance, which would tend to *increase* food intake.[43]

Ghrelin Ghrelin stimulates feeding and growth hormone release. Ghrelin is present in the hypothalamus but the main site of production is the gastric mucosa. Circulating ghrelin concentrations increase with fasting and with diet-induced weight loss in obese subjects, and are elevated in underweight, undernourished young and older subjects. In contrast, circulating concentrations decrease after ingestion of food, particularly fat and carbohydrate, and are reduced in obese people. These changes are consistent with compensatory responses to these altered nutritional states. In a recent study by the authors' group, the fasting plasma ghrelin level was found to be negatively associated with total skeletal muscle mass, but no relationship was observed with age[60] and, in general, there is no apparent change with age in circulating ghrelin concentrations. The effects of aging and undernutrition on sensitivity to ghrelin, however, have not been reported and ghrelin resistance may occur in these states. In one study, older subjects were less sensitive to the growth hormone-releasing effects of intravenous ghrelin than young adults,[61] raising the possibility that this might also be the case for its appetite-stimulating effects.

Insulin Human aging tends to be associated with increased fasting and postprandial circulating insulin concentrations.[62] These age-associated increases in insulin concentrations are due mainly to insulin resistance resulting from increased adiposity, and only to a small extent to aging itself. Furthermore, the effects of insulin per se on appetite and feeding remain unclear.

Testosterone and other androgens Circulating androgen concentrations decline with aging. This decline may contribute to the development of sarcopenia, the decrease in functional status, and reduced wellbeing that is seen in some elderly people. Although androgen replacement therapy is generally advocated for men with marked androgen deficiency, there is no consensus about its use in elderly men with less severe aging-related declines in androgen concentrations, or in elderly women. In healthy, older men with androgen deficiency, benefits have been seen in terms of muscle mass increase and, in some cases, strength.[63,64]

Two small studies have reported functional benefits when testosterone is administered in supraphysiologic doses to older, frail men. Amory and colleagues[65] gave older men with a mean total testosterone within the normal range 600 mg testosterone intramuscularly (IM), weekly for 4 weeks before elective knee replacement surgery, and found a significant increase in the ability to stand postoperatively and a trend toward improvements in walking and stair climbing, compared with placebo-treated men. Bakhshi and colleagues[66] gave older men in a rehabilitation program with low to normal testosterone levels 100 mg IM testosterone or placebo weekly, and found significant increases in grip strength and the Function Independence Measure after testosterone but not placebo.

A recent small pilot study demonstrated that in a group of undernourished community-dwelling older men and women, combined treatment with oral nutritional supplements and testosterone resulted in a reduced number of hospitalizations and number of days in hospital compared with no treatment.[67] Testosterone levels remained within physiologic limits for men in this study.

Cytokines

Cytokines are implicated in the development of anorexia, sarcopenia, and cachexia. Age-associated increases in the production or effect of satiating cytokines may contribute to the anorexia of aging.[68] Cytokines are secreted in response to significant stress, often due to malignancy or infection, or severe chronic disease.[43] Aging is often referred to as a form of stress, and is associated with increased cortisol and catecholamines.[43] The increased cortisol and catecholamine levels in turn stimulate the release of IL-6 and TNF-α.[68] Cytokines such as IL-1β, IL-6, and TNF-α are associated with anorexia.[34] Increased cytokine levels, due to the "stress" of aging per se, or the amplified stressful effects of other pathologies, may thus provide a partial explanation for the decline in appetite and body weight that occurs in many older people.[34,43]

MANAGEMENT OF UNDERNUTRITION IN OLDER PEOPLE

When an older person presents with weight loss (particularly >5%) or low BMI (particularly < 20 kg/m^2), there is a need to complete a comprehensive assessment and address the nonphysiologic factors outlined in **Box 1** when present. Often, these are not addressed and therefore no improvement is noted. Depression, in particular, is a common cause of undernutrition in the elderly. A person with depression manifesting as weight loss is unlikely to respond well to the provision of nutritional supplements only, as this does not address the loss of appetite, lack of motivation, and lack of energy usually accompanying the depression. In contrast, treating depression is likely to result in increased oral intake and increased willingness to participate in an exercise and nutrition program. Exercise is emphasized here, as weight loss often results in a loss of muscle mass and when attempting to improve nutritional health, there is a need to also focus on restoring or preserving muscle mass. A multidisciplinary approach to nutritional health is also likely to be more successful. The timely involvement of a dietitian is important. A social worker may be able to assist with finances as well as provide counseling support. An occupational therapist may be able to provide appropriate utensils in the setting of joint deformity and pain. The physiotherapist may assist with balance training and improve confidence by permitting the participation in exercise programs.

The use of the community nutritional support service is beneficial but it is important to educate that these services are used to augment nutritional intake. In Australia, for instance, the "Meals on Wheels Program" provides five main meals per week and is therefore a meal supplementation program as it cannot meet total nutritional requirements. It is not easy to manage loss of smell or taste. Safety considerations may be required, and family or carers need to be involved in terms of ensuring that the gas stove is switched off and rotten food is thrown out.[45] One recent study found that flavor intensification did not alter sensory-specific satiety.[69] However, other studies have found that the addition of flavor enhancers such as sauce to food or glutamate may be of benefit in terms of nutritional intake and therefore such strategies are worth attempting.[70–72] Eating with others should also be encouraged. In one study family-style dining, which included the ambience in the dining hall of residents being able to choose their meal and a member of staff eating with residents at the table, was compared with the control residents who chose their food 2 weeks before, had their medications dispensed during meals, and had a choice of eating in their room or in assigned seats. This study found that residents in the intervention group maintained body weight (which decreased in the control group) and increased energy intake (which decreased in the control group).[73,74] Restrictive diets should also be avoided in long-term care settings unless absolutely necessary. Liberalizing diets as opposed to the prescription of restrictive diets has been shown to enhance quality of life and food intake.[75]

Nutritional Supplements

Oral nutritional supplements such as high-energy drinks may be beneficial and it has been recommended that they are taken between meals.[76] In undernourished older people, oral nutritional supplementation has been shown by meta-analysis of controlled trials to produce weight gain, to be free of side effects, and to reduce mortality by up to 34% among patients in short-term hospital care (odds ratio 0.66 [CI 0.49–0.90]).[77,78] Effects of supplements on function are less clear as are their effects on less undernourished people, such as those living in the community, and offer up an area of research interest. Compliance is sometimes an issue as a result of diarrhea. Splitting the drink or using a lactose-free supplement may resolve this complaint. In general, older people consume too little food to meet their nutritional needs and this puts them at risk of vitamin and mineral deficiency.[79,80] Although there is no evidence to support this recommendation, there is a general belief that multivitamin supplements are beneficial in older people and they are unlikely to do harm. Calcium and vitamin D intake should be optimized. Given the changes in appetite and satiety, it has also been suggested that snacking during the day may be beneficial.[79]

Pharmacologic Therapy

The evidence supporting any pharmacologic agent for the treatment of weight loss is limited.[79] Medications trialed to date, such as mergesterol acetate, dronabinol, and human recombinant growth hormone have serious side effects especially in frail older people in whom weight loss is commonly seen, and therefore cannot be recommended for routine clinical use at this stage.

SUMMARY

Undernutrition in older people is common and presents as appetite loss or weight loss. This condition is associated with numerous adverse consequences including muscle mass loss and increasing frailty. This important health issue, an indicator of underlying nonphysiologic and physiologic changes in the individual, is frequently overlooked. A timely, comprehensive assessment is recommended including a thorough assessment of dietary intake. Addressing nonphysiologic risk factors such as depression, dementia, oral health, social isolation, iatrogenesis (medications), and poverty is important in improving nutritional health. The use of nutritional supplements is beneficial, and exercise should also be encouraged to enable restoration of muscle mass and strength. One multivitamin per day may be beneficial and most certainly will not cause harm. At present there is no convincing evidence to support pharmacologic intervention.

REFERENCES

1. Fried LP, Tangen CM, Walston J, et al. Frailty in older adults: evidence for a phenotype. J Gerontol A Biol Sci Med Sci 2001;56:M146–56.
2. Searle SD, Mitnitski A, Gahbauer EA, et al. A standard procedure for creating a frailty index. BMC Geriatr 2008;8:24.
3. Bartali B, Frongillo EA, Bandinelli S, et al. Low nutrient intake is an essential component of frailty in older persons. J Gerontol A Biol Sci Med Sci 2006;61:589–93.
4. Barone L, Milosavljevic M, Gazibarich B. Assessing the older person: is the MNA a more appropriate nutritional assessment tool than the SGA? J Nutr Health Aging 2003;7:13–7.
5. de Groot LC, Beck AM, Schroll M, et al. Evaluating the DETERMINE your nutritional health checklist and the mini nutritional assessment as tools to identify nutritional problems in elderly Europeans. Eur J Clin Nutr 1998;52:877–83.
6. Persson MD, Brismar KE, Katzarski KS, et al. Nutritional status using mini nutritional assessment and subjective global assessment predict mortality in geriatric patients. J Am Geriatr Soc 2002;50:1996–2002.
7. Saletti A, Lindgren EY, Johansson L, et al. Nutritional status according to mini nutritional assessment in an institutionalized elderly population in Sweden. Gerontology 2000;46:139–45.
8. Soini H, Routasalo P, Lagstrom H. Characteristics of the Mini-Nutritional Assessment in elderly home-care patients. Eur J Clin Nutr 2004;58:64–70.
9. Visvanathan R, Macintosh C, Callary M, et al. The nutritional status of 250 older Australian recipients of domiciliary care services and its association with outcomes at 12 months. J Am Geriatr Soc 2003;51:1007–11.
10. Chapman I, Parker B, Doran S, et al. Low-dose pramlintide reduced food intake and meal duration in healthy, normal-weight subjects. Obesity (Silver Spring) 2007;15:1179–86.
11. Beck AM, Ovesen L, Osler M. The "Mini Nutritional Assessment" (MNA) and the "Determine Your Nutritional Health" Checklist (NSI Checklist) as predictors of morbidity and mortality in an elderly Danish population. Br J Nutr 1999;81:31–6.
12. Heiat A, Vaccarino V, Krumholz HM. An evidence-based assessment of federal guidelines for overweight and obesity as they apply to elderly persons. Arch Intern Med 2001;161:1194–203.
13. Detsky AS, McLaughlin JR, Baker JP, et al. What is subjective global assessment of nutritional status? JPEN J Parenter Enteral Nutr 1987;11:8–13.
14. Guigoz Y, Lauque S, Vellas BJ. Identifying the elderly at risk for malnutrition. The Mini Nutritional Assessment. Clin Geriatr Med 2002;18:737–57.
15. Stratton RJ, King CL, Stroud MA, et al. "Malnutrition Universal Screening Tool" predicts mortality and length of hospital stay in acutely ill elderly. Br J Nutr 2006;95:325–30.
16. Wilson MM, Thomas DR, Rubenstein LZ, et al. Appetite assessment: simple appetite questionnaire predicts weight loss in community-dwelling adults and nursing home residents. Am J Clin Nutr 2005;82:1074–81.
17. Fuhrman MP, Charney P, Mueller CM. Hepatic proteins and nutrition assessment. J Am Diet Assoc 2004;104:1258–64.
18. Flegal KM, Carroll MD, Ogden CL, et al. Prevalence and trends in obesity among US adults, 1999–2000. JAMA 2002;288:1723–7.
19. Mokdad AH, Bowman BA, Ford ES, et al. The continuing epidemics of obesity and diabetes in the United States. JAMA 2001;286:1195–200.
20. Schoenborn CA, Adams PF, Barnes PM. Body weight status of adults: United States, 1997–98. Adv Data; 2002. p. 1–15.

21. Omran ML, Morley JE. Assessment of protein energy malnutrition in older persons, Part II: laboratory evaluation. Nutrition 2000;16:131–40.
22. Rumpel C, Harris TB, Madans J. Modification of the relationship between the Quetelet index and mortality by weight-loss history among older women. Ann Epidemiol 1993;3:343–50.
23. Lang IA, Llewellyn DJ, Alexander K, et al. Obesity, physical function, and mortality in older adults. J Am Geriatr Soc 2008;56:1474–8.
24. Fine JT, Colditz GA, Coakley EH, et al. A prospective study of weight change and health-related quality of life in women. JAMA 1999;282:2136–42.
25. Newman AB, Lee JS, Visser M, et al. Weight change and the conservation of lean mass in old age: the Health, Aging and Body Composition Study. Am J Clin Nutr 2005;82:872–8; quiz 915–6.
26. Villareal DT, Banks M, Siener C, et al. Physical frailty and body composition in obese elderly men and women. Obes Res 2004;12:913–20.
27. Janssen I, Mark AE. Elevated body mass index and mortality risk in the elderly. Obes Rev 2007;8:41–59.
28. Uretsky S, Messerli FH, Bangalore S, et al. Obesity paradox in patients with hypertension and coronary artery disease. Am J Med 2007;120:863–70.
29. Wannamethee SG, Shaper AG, Lennon L, et al. Decreased muscle mass and increased central adiposity are independently related to mortality in older men. Am J Clin Nutr 2007;86:1339–46.
30. Roberts SB, Fuss P, Heyman MB, et al. Control of food intake in older men. JAMA 1994;272:1601–6.
31. Chapman IM. Endocrinology of anorexia of ageing. Best Pract Res Clin Endocrinol Metab 2004;18:437–52.
32. MacIntosh C, Morley JE, Chapman IM. The anorexia of aging. Nutrition 2000;16:983–95.
33. Doherty TJ. Invited review: aging and sarcopenia. J Appl Phys 2003;95:1717–27.
34. Morley JE, Baumgartner RN. Cytokine-related aging process. J Gerontol A Biol Sci Med Sci 2004;59:M924–9.
35. Rolland Y, Czerwinski S, Abellan Van Kan G, et al. Sarcopenia: its assessment, etiology, pathogenesis, consequences and future perspectives. J Nutr Health Aging 2008;12:433–50.
36. Prentice AM, Jebb SA. Beyond body mass index. Obes Rev 2001;2:141–7.
37. Beaufrere B, Morio B. Fat and protein redistribution with aging: metabolic considerations. Eur J Clin Nutr 2000;54(Suppl 3):S48–53.
38. Cree MG, Newcomer BR, Katsanos CS, et al. Intramuscular and liver triglycerides are increased in the elderly. J Clin Endocrinol Metab 2004;89:3864–71.
39. Zamboni M, Mazzali G, Fantin F, et al. Sarcopenic obesity: a new category of obesity in the elderly. Nutr Metab Cardiovasc Dis 2008;18:388–95.
40. Potter JF, Schafer DF, Bohi RL. In-hospital mortality as a function of body mass index: an age-dependent variable. J Gerontol 1988;43:M59–63.
41. Bhasin S, Woodhouse L, Casaburi R, et al. Older men are as responsive as young men to the anabolic effects of graded doses of testosterone on the skeletal muscle. J Clin Endocrinol Metab 2005;90:678–88.
42. Mistretta CM. Anatomy and neurophysiology of the taste system in aged animals. Ann N Y Acad Sci 1989;561:277–90.
43. Chapman IM. The anorexia of aging. Clin Geriatr Med 2007;23:735–56, V.
44. Doty RL, Shaman P, Applebaum SL, et al. Smell identification ability: changes with age. Science 1984;226:1441–3.

45. Boyce JM, Shone GR. Effects of ageing on smell and taste. Postgrad Med J 2006; 82:239–41.

46. Rolls BJ, McDermott TM. Effects of age on sensory-specific satiety. Am J Clin Nutr 1991;54:988–96.

47. Clarkston WK, Pantano MM, Morley JE, et al. Evidence for the anorexia of aging: gastrointestinal transit and hunger in healthy elderly vs. young adults. Am J Phys 1997;272:R243–8.

48. Morley JE. Anorexia of aging: physiologic and pathologic. Am J Clin Nutr 1997; 66:760–73.

49. Martinez M, Hernanz A, Gomez-Cerezo J, et al. Alterations in plasma and cerebrospinal fluid levels of neuropeptides in idiopathic senile anorexia. Regul Pept 1993;49:109–17.

50. Baranowska B, Radzikowska M, Wasilewska-Dziubinska E, et al. Relationship among leptin, neuropeptide Y, and galanin in young women and in postmenopausal women. Menopause 2000;7:149–55.

51. Matsumura T, Nakayama M, Nomura A, et al. Age-related changes in plasma orexin-A concentrations. Exp Gerontol 2002;37:1127–30.

52. Kirchgessner AL. Orexins in the brain-gut axis. Endocr Rev 2002;23:1–15.

53. Beglinger C, Degen L, Matzinger D, et al. Loxiglumide, a CCK-A receptor antagonist, stimulates calorie intake and hunger feelings in humans. Am J Physiol Regul Integr Comp Physiol 2001;280:R1149–54.

54. MacIntosh CG, Morley JE, Wishart J, et al. Effect of exogenous cholecystokinin (CCK)-8 on food intake and plasma CCK, leptin, and insulin concentrations in older and young adults: evidence for increased CCK activity as a cause of the anorexia of aging. J Clin Endocrinol Metab 2001;86:5830–7.

55. Flint A, Raben A, Astrup A, et al. Glucagon-like peptide 1 promotes satiety and suppresses energy intake in humans. J Clin Invest 1998;101:515–20.

56. MacIntosh CG, Andrews JM, Jones KL, et al. Effects of age on concentrations of plasma cholecystokinin, glucagon-like peptide 1, and peptide YY and their relation to appetite and pyloric motility. Am J Clin Nutr 1999;69:999–1006.

57. Batterham RL, Cohen MA, Ellis SM, et al. Inhibition of food intake in obese subjects by peptide YY3-36. N Engl J Med 2003;349:941–8.

58. Baumgartner RN, Waters DL, Morley JE, et al. Age-related changes in sex hormones affect the sex difference in serum leptin independently of changes in body fat. Metabolism 1999;48:378–84.

59. Hislop MS, Ratanjee BD, Soule SG, et al. Effects of anabolic-androgenic steroid use or gonadal testosterone suppression on serum leptin concentration in men. Eur J Endocrinol 1999;141:40–6.

60. Tai K, Visvanathan R, Hammond AJ, et al. Fasting ghrelin is related to skeletal muscle mass in healthy adults. Eur J Nutr 2009;48:176–83.

61. Broglio F, Benso A, Castiglioni C, et al. The endocrine response to ghrelin as a function of gender in humans in young and elderly subjects. J Clin Endocrinol Metab 2003;88:1537–42.

62. Fraze E, Chiou YA, Chen YD, et al. Age-related changes in postprandial plasma glucose, insulin, and free fatty acid concentrations in nondiabetic individuals. J Am Geriatr Soc 1987;35:224–8.

63. Morley JE. Androgens and aging. Maturitas 2001;38:61–71; discussion -3.

64. Nair KS, Rizza RA, O'Brien P, et al. DHEA in elderly women and DHEA or testosterone in elderly men. N Engl J Med 2006;355:1647–59.

65. Amory JK, Chansky HA, Chansky KL, et al. Preoperative supraphysiological testosterone in older men undergoing knee replacement surgery. J Am Geriatr Soc 2002;50:1698–701.
66. Bakhshi V, Elliott M, Gentili A, et al. Testosterone improves rehabilitation outcomes in ill older men. J Am Geriatr Soc 2000;48:550–3.
67. Chapman IM, Visvanathan R, Hammond AJ, et al. Effect of testosterone and a nutritional supplement, alone and in combination, on hospital admissions in undernourished older men and women. Am J Clin Nutr 2009;89:880–9.
68. Yeh SS, Schuster MW. Geriatric cachexia: the role of cytokines. Am J Clin Nutr 1999;70:183–97.
69. Havermans RC, Geschwind N, Filla S, et al. Sensory-specific satiety is unaffected by manipulations of flavour intensity. Physiol Behav 2009.
70. Appleton KM. Increases in energy, protein and fat intake following the addition of sauce to an older person's meal. Appetite 2009;52:161–5.
71. Prescott J. Effects of added glutamate on liking for novel food flavors. Appetite 2004;42:143–50.
72. Schiffman SS, Warwick ZS. Effect of flavor enhancement of foods for the elderly on nutritional status: food intake, biochemical indices, and anthropometric measures. Physiol Behav 1993;53:395–402.
73. Nijs KA, de Graaf C, Kok FJ, et al. Effect of family style mealtimes on quality of life, physical performance, and body weight of nursing home residents: cluster randomised controlled trial. BMJ 2006;332:1180–4.
74. Nijs KA, de Graaf C, Siebelink E, et al. Effect of family-style meals on energy intake and risk of malnutrition in Dutch nursing home residents: a randomized controlled trial. J Gerontol A Biol Sci Med Sci 2006;61:935–42.
75. Womack P, Breeding C. Position of the American Dietetic Association: liberalized diets for older adults in long-term care. J Am Diet Assoc 1998;98:201–4.
76. Wilson MM, Purushothaman R, Morley JE. Effect of liquid dietary supplements on energy intake in the elderly. Am J Clin Nutr 2002;75:944–7.
77. Milne AC, Avenell A, Potter J. Meta-analysis: protein and energy supplementation in older people. Ann Intern Med 2006;144:37–48.
78. Milne AC, Potter J, Avenell A. Protein and energy supplementation in elderly people at risk from malnutrition. Cochrane Database Syst Rev 2005;CD003288.
79. Alibhai SM, Greenwood C, Payette H. An approach to the management of unintentional weight loss in elderly people. CMAJ 2005;172:773–80.
80. Wendland BE, Greenwood CE, Weinberg I, et al. Malnutrition in institutionalized seniors: the iatrogenic component. J Am Geriatr Soc 2003;51:85–90.
81. Akamizu T, Iwakura H, Ariyasu H, et al. Repeated administration of ghrelin to patients with functional dyspepsia: its effects on food intake and appetite. Eur J Endocrinol 2008;158:491–8.
82. Levin F, Edholm T, Schmidt PT, et al. Ghrelin stimulates gastric emptying and hunger in normal-weight humans. J Clin Endocrinol Metab 2006;91:3296–302.
83. Broglio F, Prodam F, Riganti F, et al. The continuous infusion of acylated ghrelin enhances growth hormone secretion and worsens glucose metabolism in humans. J Endocrinol Invest 2008;31:788–94.

Oropharyngeal Dysphagia

Ian J. Cook, MBBS, MD(Syd), FRACP

KEYWORD

- Swallow dysphagia aging treatment
  etiology pathophysiology radiography

The aging process is associated with measurable changes in nerve and muscle function. The commonest causes of pharyngeal dysphagia are neuromyogenic disorders. Although the aging process is associated with measurable changes in muscle function, aging does not usually cause pharyngeal dysphagia. However, the aging process is associated with an increased prevalence of neuromuscular disorders and systemic and degenerative processes that can be associated with or cause pharyngeal dysphagia. Hence, in the aging population, oropharyngeal dysphagia can frequently lead to severe malnutrition, aspiration, pneumonia, and death.[1] It is common in the chronic care setting, with 60% to 87% of occupants in aged care facilities having feeding difficulties,[2,3] of whom a substantial proportion have dysphagia. It is recognized that inability to feed oneself in such a setting leads to a much higher mortality rate.[4] In the general community, dysphagia is probably under-recognized in the elderly. A Dutch study reported symptomatic dysphagia in 16% of individuals older than 87 years.[5] Fibrosing disorders of the cricopharyngeus such as Zenker diverticulum, has an average age of presentation in the late ninth decade.[6] The commonest cause of dysphagia in the elderly is stroke, and this carries a high morbidity, mortality, and cost. For example, dysphagia following stroke is an independent predictor of institutionalization or subsequent hospital readmission.[7] Oropharyngeal dysphagia occurs in one third of all stroke patients.[8–10] The incidence of conditions such as Parkinson disease and Alzheimer disease increase with aging and these disorders demonstrate a 20% to 50% prevalence of oropharyngeal dysphagia.[11–13] Therapeutic response and prognosis is variable and is dependent on several factors including the underlying cause, the severity and nature of the mechanical dysfunction, and the degree of associated cognitive dysfunction when present.[14] Management of these patients generally demands a multidisciplinary approach involving the gerontologist,

Department of Gastroenterology, St George Hospital, Gray Street, Kogarah, NSW 2217, Australia
E-mail address: i.cook@unsw.edu.au

Gastroenterol Clin N Am 38 (2009) 411–431
doi:10.1016/j.gtc.2009.06.003
0889-8553/09/$ – see front matter © 2009 Published by Elsevier Inc.

gastro.theclinics.com

radiologist, gastroenterologist, neurologist, speech-language pathologist, dietician, and, at times, the palliative-care physician.

THE INFLUENCE OF THE NORMAL AGING PROCESS ON NEUROMUSCULAR FUNCTION AND ON THE OROPHARYNGEAL SWALLOW

Normal aging results in changes in nerve function, a region-dependent decline in muscle mass, and cerebral atrophy and central neuronal drop-out.[15] Age-related alterations in cortical activation are observed during swallowing.[16] This study found an increase in somatosensory cortical activation during swallowing in the elderly. The significance of this is unknown and the findings are likely to be nonspecific with an age-related increase in cortical excitability. Diffuse periventricular white matter changes apparent on MRI are believed to be related to microvascular disease in otherwise neurologically normal aged individuals. Affected individuals, not complaining of dysphagia, show prolongation of components of the swallow that correlate to a degree with the extent of such white matter changes and, if severe enough, may account for functionally significant oropharyngeal dysphagia in some cases in which the underlying cause of dysphagia is not apparent.[17,18] Concomitant medical illnesses, particularly if sufficient to require hospital admission, have been found to be associated with an increased likelihood of detecting pharyngeal dysfunction and some impairment of pharyngeal bolus clearance, even in patients who are not reporting dysphagia.[19]

Videofluoroscopic changes in the pharyngeal swallow have been reported in up to 84% of asymptomatic elderly, compared with what is considered normal in healthy young adults.[20] However, it must be appreciated that a mild increase in hypopharyngeal postswallow residue, or even age-related structural changes, are generally asymptomatic and do not necessarily lead to clinically apparent problems unless they are severe or unless they are associated with additional pathologic neuromyogenic dysfunction. For example, the cricopharyngeal bar is a common, frequently incidental radiological finding. This finding is demonstrated in 5% to 19% of patients undergoing pharyngeal videoradiography but is generally asymptomatic.[21,22] Dysphagia is no more prevalent in those individuals found to have a cricopharyngeal bar (13%) than it is in those without a bar.[22] Nonetheless, the overall duration of the oral phase[23] and the pharyngeal swallow measured radiographically is prolonged,[24] whereas the coordination among motor events measured manometrically is unaffected by normal aging.[23,25] Despite these measurable differences, the pharyngeal swallow is remarkably robust in the face of the aging process, as shown by the relative preservation of bolus clearance demonstrated scintigraphically.[26] In that study, there was no increase in bolus residue postswallow until after the age of 55 years and, even then, the pharyngeal clearance mechanism was remarkably efficient (**Fig. 1**).

There have been several manometric studies of the effects of normal aging on the upper esophageal sphincter (UES) and pharyngeal motor function. In healthy, asymptomatic elderly patients, UES resting tone is either normal or slightly reduced and UES relaxation is complete.[23,27] Peak pharyngeal contraction pressures are also preserved, or even increased, in the aged.[23,25,28] The UES in the healthy aged does show some loss of elasticity or compliance, as manifest by some reduction in sphincter opening and resulting increase in hypopharyngeal intrabolus pressure in comparison to young controls.[23]

Sensory nerve function is important for the normal swallow. Normal aging is associated with demonstrable changes in sensory function in the oral cavity and the pharynx. There is an increase in the threshold needed to trigger the pharyngeal swallow, and sensory discrimination of hypopharynx and the supraglottic structures

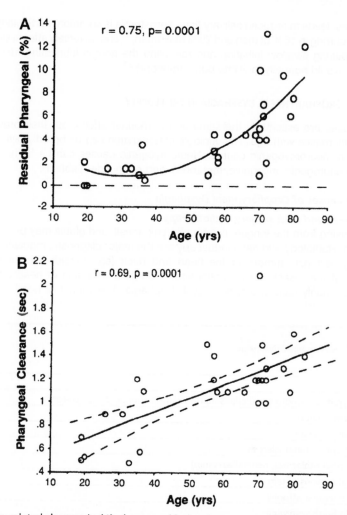

Fig. 1. Age-related changes in (*A*) pharyngeal bolus clearance and (*B*) pharyngeal clearance time, determined by pharyngeal scintigraphy during single swallows in healthy, asymptomatic, aged individuals. Note that the residual in the pharynx postswallow is remarkably low (>98% clearance) up to the age of 57 and steadily increases thereafter with advancing years. The overall pharyngeal clearance time, hence the potential laryngeal exposure time, lengthens with increasing age, which potentially exposes the individual to a greater aspiration risk, particularly if there is concurrent decompensation of other components of the swallow. (*From* Cook IJ, Weltman MD, Wallace K, et al. Influence of aging on oral-pharyngeal bolus transit and clearance during swallowing: a scintigraphic study. Am J Phys 1994;266:G972; with permission.)

is diminished in the aged.[29,30] This could render the aged pharynx more liable to aspiration in the context of additional neuromuscular dysfunction.

Age-related changes in the oral cavity can be important contributors to dysphagia in the aged. The edentulous patient can have impaired masticatory function, which can be further impaired by sarcopenia and adipose tissue replacement in the tongue, and reduced masticatory strength.[31] Aging, particularly in the context of multiple medications, leads to reduced salivary flow. Xerostomia is common, particularly in the elderly, occurring in 16% of men and 25% of women,[32] and adversely affects swallowing by impairing swallow initiation and removing the normal lubricating function of saliva that would normally facilitate bolus transport.[33]

CAUSES OF OROPHARYNGEAL DYSPHAGIA IN THE ELDERLY

These causes are essentially the same as for younger adults, but their prevalence generally increases with age. The etiologic classification can be broadly divided into structural or neuromyogenic causes. Neuromyogenic causes can be further subdivided into neurogenic, myogenic, metabolic, and endocrine (**Table 1**).

Structural Causes of Oropharyngeal Dysphagia

Tumors, head and neck surgery, radiotherapy

Tumors arising from the tongue, palate, pharynx, tonsil, and glottis may present with dysphagia. Radiology and nasoendoscopy are the major diagnostic modalities. Less commonly, extrinsic tumors of the head and neck (eg, thyroid) can also cause dysphagia if they reach a substantial size.[34] Surgical resection of head and neck cancer commonly causes oropharyngeal dysphagia. The impact of head and neck

Table 1 Causes of oropharyngeal dysphagia.
Central nervous system
Stroke
Extrapyramidal syndromes (Parkinson, Huntington chorea, Wilson disease)
Brainstem tumors
Alzheimer disease
Amyotrophic lateral sclerosis
Drugs (phenothiazines, benzodiazepines)
Peripheral nervous system
Spinal muscular atrophy
Guillain-Barré syndrome
Postpolio syndrome
Drugs (botulinum toxin, procainamide, cytotoxics)
Myogenic
Myasthenia gravis
Dermatomyositis, polymyositis, inclusion body myositis
Thryotoxic myopathy
Paraneoplastic syndromes
Drugs (amiodarone, alcohol, cholesterol-lowering drugs)
Structural disorders
Zenker diverticulum
Cricopharyngeal bar or stenosis
Cervical (mucosal) web
Oropharyngeal tumors
Head and neck surgery
Radiotherapy

cancer surgery on swallowing varies markedly among individuals and depends on many factors including the extent of surgical resection, whether flap reconstruction is required, which muscular, boney, or cartilaginous structures are removed or deranged, whether surgery causes collateral damage to neural innervation, and whether surgery is accompanied by radiotherapy, which damages muscles and nerves.[35] Because tongue base motion is so important for the generation of pharyngeal propulsive forces, the extent of tongue resection is the most important factor determining dysphagia severity in those undergoing surgery for oral cancer,[36] and the degree of preservation of tongue base motion is an important predictor of recovery of swallow function following laryngeal surgery.[37] Laryngectomy, with or without radiotherapy, can cause dysphagia due to a combination of anatomic derangements and pharyngeal muscular dysfunction.[37,38]

Radiotherapy is well recognized to cause severe nerve and muscle damage to oral and pharyngeal structures. It is not uncommon for radiation-induced dysphagia to manifest clinically more than 10 years after administration of treatment.[39] Radiation-induced xerostomia in addition is an important contributor to swallow dysfunction in the cancer patient.

Postcricoid web, cricopharyngeal bar, and stenosis

A postcricoid web is a thin, shelflike, usually eccentric but sometimes circumferential, constriction that occurs in the proximal few centimeters of the esophagus and is comprised of a thin layer of mucosa and submucosa. Webs typically present with dysphagia for solids but because of their proximal location, deglutitive aspiration may occur. One consecutive series of 1134 videofluoroscopic examinations reported a cervical esophageal web in 7.5% of unselected patients investigated for dysphagia, and were twice as common in women as in men.[40] Webs are frequently more readily appreciated on barium swallow than they are endoscopically. Inadvertent disruption of the lesion at endoscopy and a somewhat retrospective appreciation of its existence is common.

A cricopharyngeal bar is a common incidental radiological finding (see earlier discussion). Although frequently asymptomatic, it can cause function impairment to the swallow if it is associated with a Zenker diverticulum, if it is tightly stenosed, or if there is coexistent neuromyogenic disease (**Fig. 2**). Compared with appropriate disease controls without myopathy, the prevalence of the postcricoid bar is significantly more common than expected in the context of inflammatory myopathies.[41,42]

These structural lesions, when considered to be responsible for the patient's symptoms, are treated by mechanical disruption, either by cricopharyngeal myotomy or dilatation. Myotomy is most efficacious when applied to patients with structural disorders that limit opening of the cricopharyngeus in association with preserved pharyngeal contractility as seen in webs and stenoses.[43,44] Evidence supporting efficacy of either dilatation or myotomy for cervical esophageal webs and postcricoid stenosis is all uncontrolled, but consistently favorable.[45] However, repeated dilations over many years seem to be required in at least 40% of such patients and, in one study, 20% eventually required surgery.[46]

Zenker diverticulum

The posterior hypopharyngeal pouch, Zenker diverticulum, arises in the posterior hypopharyngeal wall through an area of relative muscular weakness (Killian dehiscence) just proximal to the upper margin of the cricopharyngeus muscle (**Fig. 2**). The diverticulum develops secondary to fibrosis and loss of compliance of the cricopharyngeus muscle[47] with concomitant swallow-induced increase in intrabolus flow

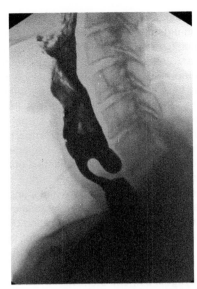

Fig. 2. Radiograph of a posterior (Zenker) diverticulum. Note the prominent postcricoid impression.

pressures just proximal to the sphincter.[6] Presenting symptoms typically include dysphagia and regurgitation. Aspiration symptoms and recurrent chest infections are common.

Cricopharyngeal myotomy, either alone or in combination with pouch resection or suspension, is the treatment of choice.[44] Myotomy can be performed either by a transcutaneous or an endoluminal approach.[48] Resection of the pouch alone is inadequate treatment and myotomy is the essential element in treatment of this condition. Simple cricopharyngeal dilatation can afford symptomatic benefit of variable duration and is a reasonable alternative in the elderly with significant comorbidity.[49–51] No controlled trials of the efficacy of surgical treatment of Zenker diverticulum exist. However, the consistency of published response rates of 80% to 100% is in keeping with the strong clinical impression that surgery is nearly always curative in this disorder.[52]

Neurogenic Causes of Oropharyngeal Dysphagia

Stroke
Stroke is the commonest cause of oropharyngeal dysphagia. Although much more common and more severe in bilateral or brainstem stroke, dysphagia affects 25% to 40% of patients in the acute phase of a unilateral hemisphere stroke.[53,54] Recent studies on the cortical topographic representation of swallow musculature in health and following hemispheric stroke have implicated hemispheric asymmetry as a determinant of dysphagia following unilateral hemisphere stroke.[55] Whether or not an individual develops dysphagia following stroke seems to be determined by the size of pharyngeal representation within the affected cortex. The degree of natural recovery of swallowing following stroke parallels the increase in size of cortical representation in the intact hemisphere. Hence, recovery of swallow function after stroke depends on the presence of intact projections from the undamaged hemisphere which, by the process of "plasticity," can develop increased control over the brainstem swallow center with time.

Of stroke patients with dysphagia, 45% to 68% are dead within 6 months largely due to dysphagia-related nutritional and pulmonary complications.[53,56] In addition to a higher mortality, dysphagia confers a higher risk of infection, poor nutrition, longer hospital stay, and institutionalization.[9,57] The most prevalent complication of stroke-related pharyngeal dysphagia is aspiration pneumonia, occurring in one third of all patients and in two thirds of those with brainstem stroke.[9] Hence, determination of the risk of aspiration in this population is a fundamental aim of management. Bedside evaluation underestimates the prevalence of deglutitive aspiration. Videofluoroscopy is vital in the assessment of aspiration risk because it can detect aspiration not evident at the time of bedside assessment in 42% to 60% of patients.[8,58] This may represent a laryngopharyngeal sensory deficit as regional mucosal sensory thresholds have been found to be increased in stroke cases, compared with controls.[59,60] If aspiration of all trialed consistencies is demonstrated, immediate introduction of nonoral feeding is indicated. Additional typical videofluoroscopic findings might include difficulty in initiating the swallow, a delayed or absent pharyngeal swallow response, pharyngeal weakness with poor pharyngeal clearance, and postswallow pooling in vallecula and pyriform sinuses. Does systematic evaluation of the stroke patient with dysphagia reduce the risk of pneumonia and influence outcome? There are no randomized controlled studies that address this question. Although the level of evidence is weak, reports of pneumonia rates from centers with dysphagia programs compared with historical data from centers without formal programs suggest that systematic evaluation by videofluoroscopy or nasoendoscopy coupled with a structured treatment program may reduce pneumonia rates.[61,62]

Parkinson disease

Dysphagia occurs commonly in Parkinson disease[11] and in related parkinsonian disorders such as dementia with Lewy bodies, corticobasal degeneration, multiple system atrophy, and progressive supranuclear palsy.[63] The median survival time from onset of dysphagia to death in these related disorders is short, ranging from 15 to 24 months.[63] The true prevalence of dysphagia in Parkinson disease is uncertain but may be as high as 52%.[64,65] Drooling of saliva is even more common than dysphagia, being reported in up to 78% of patients.[64,66] Although neither disease duration, nor severity, nor specific cardinal parkinsonian features correlate with the severity of dysphagia,[13,67,68] the latency from disease onset to onset of dysphagia correlates positively with long-term survival.[63]

Impaired preparatory lingual movements and mastication, piecemeal swallows, increased oral residue, preswallow spill, and swallow hesitancy are common radiological observations.[13,69] Lingual tremor seems to be specific for extrapyramidal movement disorders.[13,68] Intra- or postswallow aspiration occurs in one third of those with dysphagia, and silent aspiration has been reported in up to 15% of those reporting neither dysphagia nor symptoms of aspiration.[13,67]

Manometric studies may demonstrate diminished pharyngeal contraction pressures, pharyngo-sphincteric incoordination, or synchronous pressure waves, and failure of UES relaxation is common, occurring in up to 25% of cases.[13,70] Cricopharyngeal myotomy would seem to be a logical treatment in view of the high prevalence of failed UES relaxation. A favorable response to myotomy has been reported in a small series, many of whom had additional structural abnormalities, but more data are required before surgery can be recommended for the condition.[71] Unfortunately, levodopa therapy is frequently disappointing in terms of lack of favorable changes in pharyngeal mechanics dysphagia severity.[72,73] Nevertheless, evidence for a good clinical response to drug therapy exists in isolated case reports,[74] and optimal pharmacotherapy generally improves the patients' ability to feed themselves by minimizing hand tremor and bradykinesia, and treatment of mood disturbance, when present, may also improve feeding behavior and appetite. Appropriate timing of medication, 1 hour before meals, would seem logical and was found to be beneficial in at least one case report.[75] Systematic reviews of therapeutic outcome have concluded that there are no controlled data on which to base firm treatment guidelines in this disease.[76,77] However, the general principles of swallow rehabilitation applicable following stroke are generally adopted in Parkinson disease (see later discussion).

Motor neuron disease

Oropharyngeal dysphagia affects most sufferers at some stage in their disease.[78] Bulbar involvement with dysarthria and dysphagia is a primary manifestation in 25% to 30% of cases of amyotrophic lateral sclerosis.[79] The onset of the disease is insidious. Early symptoms include deglutitive cough, followed by progressive dysphagia and weight loss. The sequence of involvement of bulbar muscles is predictable in that the tongue is generally involved early and nearly always before the pharyngeal muscles. Aspiration pneumonia is a common complication, which, coupled with diminished respiratory muscle reserve, is the commonest cause of death.[80]

Videofluoroscopic findings depend on the stage of disease. By the time dysphagia is a significant problem, lingual dysfunction is almost invariably present and manifests as repetitive tongue movements, premature retrolingual bolus spill, and significant retention of barium in the oral sulci requiring several swallows for clearance. The pharyngeal swallow response may be delayed and is eventually lost with markedly impaired bolus clearance from the pharynx and intra- and postswallow aspiration of contrast. Management of these patients is difficult and necessitates involvement of the palliative care team along with institution of swallow therapy (see below), appropriately timed introduction of percutaneous endoscopic gastrostomy (PEG) feeding, and control of troublesome drooling. In addition to videofluoroscopic swallow assessments, monitoring of vital capacity and speech are useful prognostic indicators that guide the clinician as to the timing of intervention with swallow therapy and consideration of nonoral feeding.[81] However, there are no adequately controlled studies from which clear, evidence-based guidelines can dictate the optimal timing of PEG tube insertion. Whether or not early PEG placement results in increased survival or improved outcomes has not yet been demonstrated convincingly.[82] The decision is made on clinical grounds, considering a range of factors including nutritional and hydration status, aspiration risk, and patient attitude to dietary modification and the feeding process.

Centrally acting drugs causing oropharyngeal dysphagia

Drugs with dopamine antagonist action, such as phenothiazines and metoclopramide, can cause dystonia and dyskinesia resulting in dysphagia (**Table 2**). These centrally acting drugs may also impair pharyngeal propulsive and clearance functions by causing a clinical picture similar to Parkinson disease.[83] The benzodiazepines nitrazepam and clonazepam[84] have been documented to cause oropharyngeal dysphagia.

Myogenic Causes of Oropharyngeal Dysphagia

Myasthenia gravis

Dysphagia affects 30% to 60% of cases of myasthenia.[85] Dysphagia is present at diagnosis in around 20% of cases,[86] and may be the sole presenting symptom in 15% of affected individuals.[87] The so-called "fatigable flaccid dysarthria" manifested by hypernasal speech (velopharyngeal incompetence), imprecise articulation, and breathiness reflects bulbar dysfunction and is usually prominent in those with

Table 2
Drugs Associated With Oropharyngeal Dysphagia

Centrally acting drugs:
Phenothiazines[a]
Metoclopramide[a]
Benzodiazepines[a] (nitrazepam, clonazepam)
Antihistamines[a]
Drugs acting at neuromuscular junction:
Botulinum A toxin[a]
Procainamide[a]
Penicillamine
Erythromycin
Aminoglycosides
Drugs toxic to muscle:
Amiodarone[a]
Alcohol[a]
HMG-CoA reductase inhibitors[a]
Cyclosporin
Penicillamine
Miscellaneous, mechanism presumed neuromyopathic:
Digoxin[a]
Trichloroethylene[a]
Vincristine[a]
Drugs inhibiting salivation:[a]
Anticholinergics, antidepressants, antipsychotics, antihistamines, antiparkinsonian drugs, antihypertensives, diuretics

[a] Indicates that specific reports of drug-related dysphagia exist.

dysphagia; progressive difficulty chewing and swallowing during the course of a long meal may also be reported.[88] The ocular features of palpebral ptosis and diplopia are usually, but not invariably, present. Diagnosis may be apparent from typical clinical signs including fatigability, but the presentation in the elderly can be atypical, and this treatable condition should be considered in any elderly dysphagic patient even when typical ocular signs are absent.

The diagnosis is confirmed by detecting anti-acetylcholine receptor (AChR) antibodies which are present in 85% of patients.[89] The finding of AChR antibodies is highly specific and virtually diagnostic. In patients who are seronegative for AChR, and in particular those with predominant bulbar or respiratory muscle involvement, anti–muscle-specific tyrosine kinase (anti-MuSK) antibodies can be detected.[90] The edrophonium (Tensilon) stimulation test may be positive but single-fiber electromyographic (EMG) recording is the most sensitive diagnostic test.[85]

The response of pharyngeal swallow dysfunction to an acetylcholinesterase inhibitor and immunosuppressive therapy is variable and may respond less satisfactorily than do other muscle groups. Even in those with a satisfactory clinical response, the videofluoroscopic improvement following therapy may be marginal, which casts doubt on the use of videofluoroscopy in assessing the progress of these patients.[88] Notwithstanding the frequently disappointing response to medical therapy, establishing the diagnosis does influence management as it always warrants drug therapy, a search for thymoma, and avoidance of risk factors for myasthenic crisis, to which the dysphagic patient is frequently exposed, including respiratory tract infections, anesthesia, and surgery.

Inflammatory myopathies

Dysphagia complicates 30% to 60% of cases of inflammatory myopathy (polymyositis, dermatomyositis, and inclusion body myositis).[85,91] The clinical features of inflammatory myopathy generally include a subacute or chronic and progressive symmetric, proximal, muscular weakness. However, one third of those affected presenting with dysphagia as their only presenting symptom will have no clinically apparent extrabulbar muscular weakness.[42]

Diagnosis maybe confirmed by abnormalities of one or more of muscle enzymes, EMG, or muscle biopsy. Serum creatine phosphokinase (CPK) is the most sensitive enzyme but the CPK level is normal, even in active disease, and in 25% of those with dysphagia as their presenting complaint.[42,91] Electromyography is useful in excluding neurogenic disorders and will demonstrate features consistent with inflammatory myositis in 85% to 90%.[92] Muscle biopsy is required for definitive diagnosis and to distinguish between dermatomyositis, polymyositis, and inclusion body myositis. Notwithstanding, muscle biopsy is diagnostic in only 80%, emphasizing that diagnosis of myositis can be elusive and the need for complete clinical, biochemical, and laboratory evaluation in suspected cases.[42,92] The inflammatory process may be patchy and is occasionally confined to the pharyngeal musculature.[93]

The videofluoroscopic features are variable. Pharyngeal dysfunction is almost invariably present and radiographic evidence of aspiration is seen in 60%.[94] Restrictive cricopharyngeal disorders (cricopharyngeal bar, cricopharyngeal stenosis, and Zenker) are more commonly seen in inflammatory myopathy presenting with dysphagia than they are in neurogenic dysphagia.[42] Combined videoradiographic and manometric evaluation of this population showed normal sphincter relaxation, restricted sphincter opening, and raised hypopharyngeal intrabolus pressures (**Fig. 3**).

The mainstay of treatment of inflammatory myopathies is immunosuppressive therapy with steroids in the first instance, with azathioprine or methotrexate as second line or steroid-sparing agents. Despite the lack of controlled efficacy trials, a significant number of patients respond favorably to these agents. High-dose intravenous immunoglobulin has been shown to be of clear benefit in a controlled trial for those with polymyositis and dermatomyositis, although inclusion body myositis is generally resistant to standard therapies.[95] Given the common finding of restricted UES opening in this population, cricopharyngeal disruption can be beneficial in at least 50% of patients.[96]

Toxic and metabolic myopathies

Muscle weakness affects 80% of thyrotoxic patients and men are affected more commonly than women.[97] Associated pharyngeal dysphagia is generally slowly progressive and may be the presenting feature of this endocrinopathy.[98] Although uncommon, this condition should always be considered, particularly in the elderly when the more classic thyrotoxic features may be absent, because it is a reversible cause of dysphagia. The pharyngeal dysphagia usually responds well to treatment with restoration of the euthyroid state.[98] Several drugs capable of causing toxic or inflammatory myopathy should be considered in the assessment of the patient with dysphagia, as removal of the drug generally reverses the dysphagia (**Table 2**).

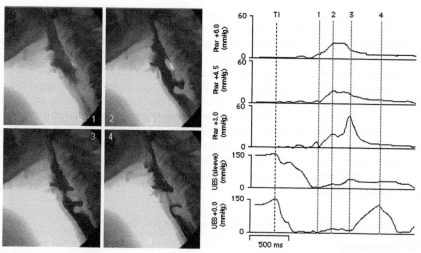

Fig. 3. Videoradiographic sequence (*left*) and corresponding manometry in a patient with myositis, a cricopharyngeal bar, and early diverticulum. Note the poor pharyngeal bolus clearance from a combination of pharyngeal weakness and restrictive defect at the UES. Each vertical dashed line represents the time corresponding to the numbered radiographic frame on the left. Note that the sphincter relaxes completely and there is a pharyngeal swallow response detected radiographically and manometrically. Although the pharyngeal stripping wave is apparent, it is of low amplitude. Hypopharyngeal intrabolus pressure (*frame 2, channel 3*) is increased due to the marked restriction in sphincter opening. TI, onset of swallow indicated by initial tongue tip motion at the maxillary incisors. (*From* Williams RB, Grehan MJ, Hersch M, et al. Biomechanics, diagnosis, and treatment outcome in inflammatory myopathy presenting as oropharyngeal dysphagia. Gut 2003;52:471; with permission.)

Presenting Features and Clinical Assessment of Oropharyngeal Dysphagia

Oropharyngeal dysphagia can manifest with one or more symptoms that are specific for oropharyngeal dysfunction and which help the clinician distinguish it from esophageal dysphagia. Swallow initiation may be delayed or absent. Aspiration may manifest as deglutitive cough. Nasopharyngeal regurgitation may be reported. Excessive postswallow residue commonly necessitates repeated swallows to effect pharyngeal clearance. The patient may describe the bolus holding up in the neck but this can be a false localizing feature of esophageal dysphagia and is certainly not specific for pharyngeal dysfunction. It is usual for several of these symptoms to manifest simultaneously in the dysphagic patient. In addition, in the aged population, weight loss, nutritional deficiency, and pneumonia are not uncommon presenting problems.

The circumstances of symptom onset, duration, and progression of dysphagia provide useful diagnostic information. A sudden onset of dysphagia, often in association with other neurologic symptoms or signs, usually indicates a cerebrovascular event. A more insidious onset is more consistent with disorders such as inflammatory myopathy, myasthenia, or amyotrophic lateral sclerosis. Additional neurologic symptoms, when present, such as vertigo, nausea, vomiting, hiccup, hoarseness, tinnitus, diplopia, and so forth, may help localize a lesion to the brainstem. More widespread neuromuscular symptoms such as dysarthria, diplopia, limb weakness, or fatigability might suggest a motor neuronal or myopathic etiology.

The elderly patient with oropharyngeal dysphagia needs a careful neurologic assessment. The diagnostic workup of these patients aims to: (1) identify features of underlying systemic or metabolic disease when present; (2) localize, if possible, the neuroanatomical level and severity of a causative neurologic lesion when present; and (3) detect adverse sequelae such as pulmonary sepsis or nutritional deficiency, which are important indicators of the severity of dysphagia. In addition, an assessment by a speech-language pathologist will provide further information about language, cognitive and behavioral dysfunction, as well as the strength and range of movement of the muscles involved in speech and swallowing. This information will directly influence decisions as to the patient's suitability for swallow therapy and the type of therapy adopted. An important role of the speech pathologist is to conduct a videofluoroscopic swallow study, usually called a modified barium swallow, to assess aspiration risk and to guide therapy.

Techniques to Evaluate the Patient with Oropharyngeal Dysphagia

Videofluoroscopy
Static films, obtained during a standard barium swallow, may provide important clues to the presence of pharyngeal neuromuscular dysfunction, such as impaired pharyngeal clearance and tracheal aspiration (**Fig. 4**). A standard barium swallow can readily identify structural causes of dysphagia such as diverticula, webs, stenoses, or cancers. However, static films are inadequate to define the mechanics of the abnormal swallow, which is achieved by performing a modified barium swallow.[99] This test

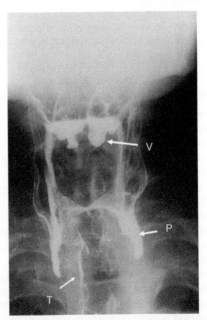

Fig. 4. Barium radiograph of the pharynx immediately following the swallow. Although the optimal way to detect pharyngeal dysfunction is with a videoswallow, important clues to pharyngeal dysfunction can be obtained from spot films such as this. The excess pooling of contrast in the vallucula (V) and pyriform sinuses (P) indicates impaired clearance due to pharyngeal weakness. The postswallow contrast within the trachea (T) indicates aspiration.

acquires dedicated lateral and anteroposterior views of the oral and pharyngeal phases of the swallow, permits standard and slow motion replay of the swallow to define the mechanisms and severity of dysfunction as well as the influence of modifications to bolus consistency, postures and other swallow maneuvers on bolus flow and clearance. Videofluoroscopy is a sensitive means of confirming oral-pharyngeal dysfunction if its presence is uncertain on the basis of history. This technique provides information on the presence and severity of the major categories of dysfunction, including the presence, timing, and severity of aspiration. Identification of these mechanisms assists the therapist in deciding on specific swallow therapies and the need for nonoral feeding when aspiration is demonstrated.

Nasoendoscopy

Fiberoptic nasoendoscopy is the optimal method for identifying mucosal abnormalities and choosing the site for biopsy, and is mandatory in all cases in which malignancy is suspected. Nasoendoscopy, frequently referred to as fiberoptic endoscopic examination of swallowing (FEES), is less well suited to the assessment of swallow mechanics than videofluoroscopy but can detect the absence of, or profound delay in, initiating the pharyngeal swallow response, and can provide indirect evidence of aspiration.[100]

Manometry

Intraluminal manometry can quantify pharyngeal deglutitive forces, detect failure of UES relaxation, and the relative coordination of pharyngeal contraction with UES relaxation.[13,101–103] The age-related changes in manometric parameters dictate the need for comparison with appropriate normative values.[23,104] It is often useful to combine manometry with videofluoroscopy. This technique permits correlation of the motion of anatomic structures with the resulting intraluminal pressures[105,106] and the identification of intrabolus pressure, which is an indirect measure of UES compliance.[6] Failure of UES relaxation, which can only be reliably determined by manometry or EMG, indicates a rostral medullary lesion or Parkinson disease.[13,107,108] Identification of certain manometric abnormalities, particularly failed UES relaxation or elevated intrabolus pressure, may help in diagnosis and may influence management decisions, particularly relating to the advisability of cricopharyngeal myotomy or dilatation.[13,102,109,110] However, it remains to be proven that such intervention in this context influences clinical outcome.

Management of Oropharyngeal Dysphagia

Management principles

Broadly speaking, the aims of management are to identify and treat an underlying primary disease if possible, and then try to compensate for or circumvent the specific mechanical disturbances responsible for the dysphagia and to eliminate or minimize aspiration if present.[14]

First, confirm that oropharyngeal dysphagia is indeed a problem and attempt to identify the underlying cause. A careful history will generally distinguish oropharyngeal dysphagia from globus, xerostomia, and esophageal dysphagia. History and physical examination may provide clues of a treatable systemic, metabolic, or drug-related disorder. This examination should include a "dysphagia screen" of laboratory tests to exclude systemic, metabolic, or directly treatable neuromyogenic diseases (eg, thyrotoxicosis, myasthenia, myositis). This laboratory screen includes CPK, erythrocyte sedimentation rate (ESR), thyroid function tests, and AChR antibodies (and, if negative, MuSK antibodies; see earlier). A cerebral MRI or CT scan is frequently indicated if a cerebrovascular event is suspected.

Second, identify the structural or neuromyogenic mechanisms of oropharyngeal dysfunction. Structural disorders are generally readily detected by radiographic or endoscopic evaluation. Identification of a neoplasm or a Zenker diverticulum will dictate surgery. A cervical web or a cricopharyngeal stenosis will prompt dilatation or, in some cases, cricopharyngeal myotomy. Nasoendoscopic examination of the laryngopharynx is mandatory if neoplasm is suspected. In the context of disorders with a high prevalence of failed UES relaxation, such as Parkinson disease and medullary lesions, pharyngeal manometry, with or without concurrent videofluoroscopy, may detect failed UES relaxation, which might prompt consideration for cricopharyngeal myotomy.

Third, determine the risk of aspiration pneumonia, which is the primary factor in the decision as to whether and when nonoral feeding should be instituted. The risk of aspiration is best determined by the modified barium swallow examination, as this risk is underestimated by about 50% by clinical assessment alone.[111] The decision on the advisability of gastrostomy feeding is also influenced by the likelihood that therapeutic maneuvers, which may be tested during videofluoroscopy, will reduce or eliminate aspiration; the natural history of the underlying disease; and the patient's cognitive ability.[7]

Finally, after exclusion of structural lesions and underlying treatable diseases, and having established the safety of oral feeding, specific "local" therapy should be considered. The therapeutic options open are dietary modification, swallow therapy, or surgery, or a combination of all three.

Dietary modification and swallow therapy

Therapeutic strategies include dietary modification, manipulation of swallowing posture, or swallowing technique. Modifications of swallowing technique are intended to strengthen weak oropharyngeal muscle groups, thereby improving their speed and range of movement, or to selectively modify the mechanics of the swallow to facilitate bolus flow and minimize aspiration. In applying swallow therapies the speech-language pathologist will use videofluoroscopy to define the relevant mechanism of dysfunction and examine the acute effects of therapeutic strategies designed to eliminate or compensate for that dysfunction.[99] Simple dietary modification has been shown in a single, randomized, controlled trial to reduce the risk of aspiration pneumonia, and should be instituted if an aspiration risk is apparent.[58] Most of the studies in this field have focused on poststroke dysphagia. There are reasonable data supporting the biologic plausibility of the remaining swallow strategies, but the limited available controlled efficacy data are inconclusive.[14,112] There is only one published randomized controlled trial of swallow behavioral therapy.[113] Twelve months after acute stroke, 15% of that study population developed one or more of the study end points, thus failing to show benefit for intensive swallow rehabilitation. On the other hand, swallow therapy has not been proven to be ineffective, and, based on the demonstration of biologic plausibility for specific therapeutic techniques, the consistency of the low grade evidence suggesting efficacy, the low cost, and the absence of either risk or any better alternative in many instances, it is appropriate to institute swallow therapy under the supervision of a speech-language pathologist. Large-scale controlled trials are necessary to clarify the appropriateness of all current treatment strategies in neurogenic oropharyngeal dysphagia.

Enteral tube feeding

PEG tubes, or nasogastric tubes (NGTs), are frequently used to feed stroke patients enterally to prevent or minimize the risk of aspiration pneumonia. There are five studies comparing the two techniques.[114–117] Whereas PEG seems to be superior in terms of reliable delivery of prescribed calories, PEG was not found to be superior to NGT in preventing aspiration, in reducing mortality, nor poor outcome at 6 months in dysphagic patients following stroke. Of some concern, the largest prospective randomized controlled trial, comparing PEG with NGT feeding, found PEG feeding to be associated with a 7% higher risk of death or poor outcome at 6 months.[117] On the basis of available evidence, a reasonable approach in patients with stroke-related dysphagia who have aspiration demonstrated radiographically on all bolus consistencies trialed, is to place an NGT in the first instance. Because of the substantial spontaneous recovery rate following stroke, if the NGT is well tolerated, and if the patient does not habitually remove the tube, then the swallow function and aspiration risk can be re-evaluated by repeat modified barium swallow in 3 to 4 weeks. If the aspiration risk persists, the NGT can be replaced by a PEG tube. This recommendation may need to be modified on a case-by-case basis and under specific circumstances. For example, hospital and nursing policies vary greatly among specific rehabilitation and aged care facilities. Unfortunately, in some cases these policies are not evidence-based but are driven by health economics.

Surgical options

The indications for surgery for structural abnormalities are discussed above. Surgical approaches may be considered in neuromyogenic dysphagia if time-related recovery or treatment of specific neuromyogenic disease has been disappointing. Several indicators have been proposed that might predict a favorable outcome from cricopharyngeal myotomy, such as: intact swallow initiation, "adequate" lingual and pharyngeal propulsive forces, radiographic or manometric evidence of increased outflow resistance at the UES (failed relaxation or constriction), and a good prognosis for the underlying neurologic disease.[109,118] Although the data supporting the efficacy of cricopharyngeal myotomy for structural cricopharyngeal disorders are strong, the outcome following myotomy for neuromyogenic dysphagia is far less certain. There are no controlled trials of cricopharyngeal myotomy in neurogenic dysphagia, but the available evidence suggests an overall response rate of around 60% with an operative mortality of 1% to 2%.[119,120]

Most surgical procedures in the dysphagic patient aim to reduce or eliminate aspiration.[121] The more conservative procedures (laryngeal suspension, vocal fold augmentation or medialization, and epiglottoplasty) preserve voice. The more destructive procedures, which achieve tracheo-esophageal separation, render the patient unable to phonate. Such procedures include glottic closure, tracheo-esophageal diversion, laryngotracheal separation, and total laryngectomy. There is virtually no reliable efficacy data on which to base recommendations and indications for such therapies.

Botulinum toxin injection

Botox injection, either endoscopically or transcutaneously, has been reported in small case series to be of benefit.[122] Although these studies attempted to target cricopharyngeal disorders, optimal identification of failed cricopharyngeal relaxation was not adopted in those studies. Diffusion of the toxin to adjacent muscles may worsen dysphagia or cause vocal-cord dysfunction. Controlled trials of the safety and efficacy of Botox is required before it might be used to target particular dysphagic populations.

REFERENCES

1. Tibbling L, Gustafsson B. Dysphagia and its consequences in the elderly. Dysphagia 1991;6:200.
2. Groher ME. The prevalence of swallowing disorders in two teaching hospitals. Dysphagia 1986;1:3.
3. Steele CM, Greenwood C, Ens I, et al. Mealtime difficulties in a home for the aged: not just dysphagia. Dysphagia 1997;12:43.
4. Siebens H, Trupe E, Siebens A, et al. Correlates and consequences of eating dependency in institutionalized elderly. J Am Geriatr Soc 1986;34:192.
5. Bloem B, Lagaay A, van Beek W, et al. Prevalence of subjective dysphagia in community residents aged over 87. Br Med J 1990;300:721.
6. Cook IJ, Gabb M, Panagopoulos V, et al. Pharyngeal (Zenker's) diverticulum is a disorder of upper esophageal sphincter opening. Gastroenterology 1992; 103:1229.
7. Smithard DG, O'Neill PA, England RE, et al. The natural history of dysphagia following a stroke. Dysphagia 1997;12:188.
8. Horner J, Massey EW, Riski JE, et al. Aspiration following stroke: clinical correlates and outcome. Neurology 1988;38:1359.
9. Young EC, Durant-Jones L. Developing a dysphagia program in an acute care hospital: a needs assessment. Dysphagia 1990;5:159.
10. Gordon C, Hewer RL, Wade DT. Dysphagia in acute stroke. Br Med J 1987;295:411.
11. Edwards LL, Eamonn BS, Quigley MM, et al. Gastrointestinal dysfunction in Parkinson's disease: frequency and pathophysiology. Neurology 1992;42:726.
12. Horner J, Alberts MJ, Dawson DV, et al. Swallowing in Alzheimer's disease. Alzheimer Dis Assoc Disord 1994;8:177.
13. Ali GN, Wallace KL, Schwartz R, et al. Mechanisms of oral-pharyngeal dysphagia in patients with Parkinson's disease. Gastroenterology 1996;110:383.
14. Cook IJ, Kahrilas PJ. American gastroenterological association technical review on management of oropharyngeal dysphagia. Gastroenterology 1999;116:455.
15. Masoro E. Biology of aging. Arch Intern Med 1987;147:166.
16. Teismann IK, Steinstraeter O, Schwindt W, et al. Age-related changes in cortical swallowing processing. Neurobiol Aging 2008.
17. Levine R, Robbins J, Maser A. Periventricular white matter changes and oropharyngeal swallowing in normal individuals. Dysphagia 1992;7:142.
18. Buchholz DW. Neurogenic dysphagia: what is the cause when the cause is not obvious? Dysphagia 1994;9:245.
19. Kendall KA, Leonard RJ, McKenzie S. Common medical conditions in the elderly: impact on pharyngeal bolus transit. Dysphagia 2004;19:71.
20. Ekberg O, Feinberg MJ. Altered swallowing function in elderly patients without dysphagia: radiographic findings in 56 patients. AJR Am J Roentgenol 1991; 156:1181.
21. Ekberg O, Nylander B. Dysfunction of the cricopharyngeal muscle. Radiology 1982;143:481.
22. Curtis DJ, Cruess DF, Berg T. The cricopharyngeal muscle: a videorecording review. AJR Am J Roentgenol 1984;142:497.
23. Shaw DW, Cook IJ, Gabb M, et al. Influence of normal aging on oral-pharyngeal and upper esophageal sphincter function during swallowing. Am J Phys 1995; 268:G389.
24. Robbins J, Hamilton JW, Lof GL, et al. Oropharyngeal swallowing in normal adults of different ages. Gastroenterology 1992;103:823.

25. Wilson J, Pryde A, Macintyre C, et al. The effects of age, sex, and smoking on normal pharyngoesophageal motility. Am J Gastroenterol 1990;85:686.
26. Cook IJ, Weltman MD, Wallace K, et al. Influence of aging on oral-pharyngeal bolus transit and clearance during swallowing: a scintigraphic study. Am J Phys 1994;266:G972.
27. Fulp SR, Dalton CB, Castell JA, et al. Aging-related alterations in human upper esophageal sphincter function. Am J Gastroenterol 1990;85:1569.
28. Shaker R, Ren J, Podvrsan B, et al. Effect of aging and bolus variables on pharyngeal and upper esophageal sphincter motor function. Am J Phys 1993; 264:G427.
29. Shaker R, Ren J, Zamir Z, et al. Effect of aging, position, and temperature on the threshold volume triggering pharyngeal swallows. Gastroenterology 1994;107: 396.
30. Aviv JE, Martin JH, Jones ME, et al. Age-related changes in pharyngeal and supraglottic sensation. Ann Otol Rhinol Laryngol 1994;103:749.
31. Rother P, Wohlgemuth B, Wolff W, et al. Morphometrically observable aging changes in the human tongue. Ann Anat 2002;184:159.
32. Rhodus NL, Moller K, Colby S, et al. Dysphagia in patients with three different etiologies of salivary gland dysfunction. Ear Nose Throat J 1995;74:39.
33. Heeneman H, Brown D. Senescent changes in and about the oral cavity and pharynx. J Otolaryngol 1986;15:214.
34. Van Ruiswyk J, Cunningham C, Cerletty J. Obstructive manifestations of thyroid lymphoma. Arch Intern Med 1989;149:1575.
35. Walther EK. Dysphagia after pharyngolaryngeal cancer surgery. Part 1: pathophysiology of postsurgical deglutition. Dysphagia 1995;10:275.
36. McConnel FM, Logemann JA, Rademaker AW, et al. Surgical variables affecting postoperative swallowing efficiency in oral cancer patients: a pilot study. Laryngoscope 1994;104:87.
37. Logemann JA, Gibbons P, Rademaker AW, et al. Mechanisms of recovery of swallow after supraglottic laryngectomy. J Speech Hear Res 1994;37:965.
38. Maclean J, Cotton S, Perry A. Post-laryngectomy: it's hard to swallow: an Australian study of prevalence and self-reports of swallowing function after a total laryngectomy. Dysphagia 2008.
39. Shapiro BE, Rordorf G, Schwamm L, et al. Delayed radiation-induced bulbar palsy. Neurology 1996;46:1604.
40. Ekberg O, Malmquist J, Lindgren S. Pharyngo-oesophageal webs in dysphageal patients. A radiologic and clinical investigation in 1134 patients. Rofo 1986;145:75.
41. Georgalas C, Baer ST. Pharyngeal pouch and polymyositis: association and implications for aetiology of Zenker's diverticulum. J Laryngol Otol 2000;114: 805.
42. Williams RB, Grehan MJ, Hersch M, et al. Biomechanics, diagnosis, and treatment outcome in inflammatory myopathy presenting as oropharyngeal dysphagia. Gut 2003;52:471.
43. Lindgren S, Ekberg O. Cricopharyngeal myotomy in the treatment of dysphagia. Clin Otolaryngol 1990;15:221.
44. Jamieson GG, Duranceau AC, Payne WS. Pharyngo-oesophageal diverticulum. In: Jamieson GG, editor. Surgery of the oesophagus. Edinburgh: Churchill Livingstone Press; 1988. p. 435.
45. Solt J, Bajor J, Moizs M, et al. Primary cricopharyngeal dysfunction: treatment with balloon catheter dilatation. Gastrointest Endosc 2001;54:767.

46. Lindgren S. Endoscopic dilatation and surgical myectomy of symptomatic cervical esophageal webs. Dysphagia 1991;6:235.

47. Cook IJ, Blumbergs P, Cash K, et al. Structural abnormalities of the cricopharyngeus muscle in patients with pharyngeal (Zenker's) diverticulum. J Gastroenterol Hepatol 1992;7:556.

48. Collard JM, Otte JB, Kestens PJ. Endoscopic stapling technique for esophagodiverticulostomy for Zenker's diverticulum. Ann Thorac Surg 1993;56:573.

49. Negus VE. The etiology of pharyngeal diverticula. Bull Johns Hopkins Hosp 1957;100:209.

50. Crescenzo DG, Trastek VF, Allen MS, et al. Zenker's diverticulum in the elderly: is operation justified? Ann Thorac Surg 1998;66:347.

51. Wang AY, Kadkade R, Kahrilas PJ, et al. Effectiveness of esophageal dilation for symptomatic cricopharyngeal bar. Gastrointest Endosc 2005;61:148.

52. Lerut T, Van Raemdonck D, Guelinckx P. Pharyngo-oesophageal diverticulum (Zenker's). Clinical therapeutic and morphological aspects. Acta Gastroenterol Belg 1990;53:330.

53. Barer DH. The natural history and functional consequence of dysphagia after hemisphere stroke. J Neurol Neurosurg Psychiatr 1989;52:236.

54. Gresham SL. Clinical assessment and management of swallowing difficulties after stroke. Med J Aust 1990;153:397.

55. Hamdy S, Aziz Q, Rothwell JC, et al. The cortical topography of human swallowing musculature in health and disease [see comments]. Nat Med 1996;2:1217.

56. Schmidt J, Holas M, Halvorson K, et al. Videofluoroscopic evidence of aspiration predicts pneumonia and death but not dehydration following stroke. Dysphagia 1994;9:7.

57. Smithard DG, O'Neill PA, Park C, et al. Complications and outcome after acute stroke: does dysphagia matter? [Published erratum appears in Stroke 1998 Jul;29(7):1480-1]. Stroke 1996;27:1200–4.

58. Groher ME. Bolus management and aspiration pneumonia in patients with pseudobulbar dysphagia. Dysphagia 1987;1:215.

59. Aviv JE, Sacco RL, Thomson J, et al. Silent laryngopharyngeal sensory deficits after stroke. Ann Otol Rhinol Laryngol 1997;106:87.

60. Mann G, Hankey GJ, Cameron D. Swallowing function after stroke. Prognosis and prognostic factors at six months. Stroke 1999;30:744.

61. Daniels SK, Brailey K, Preistly DH, et al. Aspiration in patients with acute stroke. Arch Phys Med Rehabil 1998;79:14.

62. Doggett DL, Tappe KA, Mitchell MD, et al. Prevention of pneumonia in elderly stroke patients by systematic diagnosis and treatment of dysphagia: an evidence-based comprehensive analysis of the literature. Dysphagia 2001;16:279.

63. Muller J, Wenning GK, Verny M, et al. Progression of dysarthria and dysphagia in postmortem-confirmed parkinsonian disorders. Arch Neurol 2001;58:259.

64. Edwards LL, Pfeiffer RF, Quigley EMM, et al. Gastrointestinal symptoms in Parkinson's disease. Mov Disord 1991;6:151.

65. Kuhlemeier KV. Epidemiology and dysphagia [Review]. Dysphagia 1994;9:209.

66. Johnston BT, Li Q, Castell JA, et al. Swallowing and esophageal function in Parkinson's disease. Am J Gastroenterol 1995;90:1741.

67. Robbins J, Logemann J, Kirshner H. Swallowing and speech production in Parkinson's disease. Ann Neurol 1986;19:283.

68. Edwards LL, Quigley EM, Harned RK, et al. Characterization of swallowing and defecation in Parkinson's disease. Am J Gastroenterol 1994;89:15.

69. Leopold NA, Kagel MC. Prepharyngeal dysphagia in Parkinson's disease. Dysphagia 1996;11:14.
70. Hurwitz AL, Nelson JA, Haddad JK. Oropharyngeal dysphagia: manometric and cine-esophagographic findings. Am J Dig Dis 1975;20:313.
71. Born LJ, Harned RH, Rikkers LF, et al. Cricopharyngeal dysfunction in Parkinson's disease: role in dysphagia and response to myotomy. Mov Disord 1996; 11:53.
72. Bushmann M, Dobmeyer SM, Leeker L, et al. Swallowing abnormalities and their response to treatment in Parkinson's disease. Neurology 1989;39:1309.
73. Hunter PC, Crameri J, Austin S, et al. Response of parkinsonian swallowing dysfunction to dopaminergic stimulation. J Neurol Neurosurg Psychiatr 1997; 63:579.
74. Thomas M, Haigh RA. Dysphagia, a reversible cause not to be forgotten. Postgrad Med J 1995;71:94.
75. Fonda D, Schwarz J, Clinnick S. Parkinsonian medication one hour before meals improves symptomatic swallowing: a case study. Dysphagia 1995;10:165.
76. El-Sharkawi AL, Ramig L, Logemann JA, et al. Voice treatment (LSVT) and swallowing in Parkinson's disease. Mov Disord 1998;13:121 (Abstract).
77. Deane KH, Whurr R, Clarke CE, et al. Non-pharmacological therapies for dysphagia in Parkinson's disease (Cochrane review), in Cochrane Database Syst Rev. Oxford, 2002, Vol Issue 1. p. CD002816.
78. Mayberry JF, Atkinson M. Swallowing problems in patients with motor neuron disease. J Clin Gastroenterol 1986;8:233.
79. Tandan R, Bradley WG. Amyotrophic lateral sclerosis: part I: clinical features, pathology, and ethical issues in management. Ann Neurol 1985;18:271.
80. Mulder DW. The diagnosis and treatment of amyotrophic lateral sclerosis. Boston (MA): Houghton Mifflin; 1980.
81. Strand EA, Miller RM, Yorkston KM, et al. Management of oral-pharyngeal dysphagia symptoms in amyotrophic lateral sclerosis. Dysphagia 1996;11:129.
82. Chio A, Finocchiaro E, Meineri P, et al. Safety and factors related to survival after percutaneous endoscopic gastrostomy in ALS. ALS Percutaneous Endoscopic Gastrostomy Study Group. Neurology 1999;53:1123.
83. Leopold NA. Dysphagia in drug-induced parkinsonism: a case report. Dysphagia 1996;11:151.
84. Buchholz D, Jones B, Neumann W, et al. Two cases of benzodiazepine induced pharyngeal dysphagia (abstract). McLean, Virginia: Proc Dysphagia Res Society Conference; 1994.
85. Dumitru D. Electrodiagnostic medicine. Philadelphia: Hanley and Belfus, Inc; 1995.
86. Osserman KE, Genkins G. Studies in myasthenia gravis: review of a 20 year experience in over 1200 patients. Mt Sinai J Med 1971;38:497.
87. Sanders DB, Howard JF, Disorders of neuromuscular transmission. In: Bradley WG, Daroff RB, Fenichel GM, et al, editors. Neurology in clinical practice, vol. 2, 1st edition. Massachusetts: Butterworth, Heinemann, 1991. p. 1819
88. Kluin KJ, Bromberg MB, Feldman EL, et al. Dysphagia in elderly men with myasthenia gravis. J Neurol Sci 1996;138:49.
89. Newson-Davis J. Myasthenia gravis and related syndromes. In: Walton J, Karpati G, Hilton-Jones D, editors. Disorders of voluntary muscle. 6th edition. Edinburgh: Churchill Livingstone; 1994. p. 761.
90. Evoli A, Tonali PA, Padua L, et al. Clinical correlates with anti-MuSK antibodies in generalized seronegative myasthenia gravis. Brain 2003;126:2304.

91. Dalakas MC. Polymyositis, dermatomyosotis and inclusion body myositis. N Engl J Med 1991;325:1487.
92. Tymms KE, Webb J. Dermatopolymyositis and other connective tissue diseases: a review of 105 cases. J Rheumatol 1985;12:1140.
93. Shapiro J, Martin S, DeGirolami U, et al. Inflammatory myopathy causing pharyngeal dysphagia: a new entity. Ann Otol Rhinol Laryngol 1996;105:331.
94. Johnson ER, McKenzie SW. Kinematic pharyngeal transit times in myopathy: evaluation for dysphagia. Dysphagia 1993;8:35.
95. Dalakas MC, Illa I, Dambrosia JM, et al. A controlled trial of high dose intravenous immune globulin infusions as treatment of dermatomyositis. N Engl J Med 1993;329:1993.
96. Darrow DH, Hoffman GT, Barnes GJ, et al. Management of dysphagia in inclusion body myositis. Arch Otolaryngol Head Neck Surg 1992;118:313.
97. Walton J, Karpati G, Hilton-Jones D. Disorders of voluntary muscle. 6th edition. Edinburgh: Churchill Livingstone; 1994.
98. Branski D, Levy J, Globus M, et al. Dysphagia as a primary manifestation of hyperthyroidism. J Clin Gastroenterol 1984;6:437.
99. Logemann JA. Role of the modified barium swallow in management of patients with dysphagia. Otolaryngol Head Neck Surg 1997;116:335.
100. Murray J, Langmore SE, Ginsberg S, et al. The significance of accumulated oropharyngeal secretions and swallowing frequency in predicting aspiration. Dysphagia 1996;11:99.
101. Castell J, Dalton C, Castell D. Pharyngeal and upper esophageal sphincter manometry in humans. Am J Phys 1990;258:G173.
102. Cook IJ. Cricopharyngeal function and dysfunction. Dysphagia 1993;8:244.
103. Olsson R, Castell JA, Castell DO, et al. Solid-state computerized manometry improves diagnostic yield in pharyngeal dysphagia: simultaneous videoradiography and manometry in dysphagia patients with normal barium swallows. Abdom Imaging 1995;20:230.
104. Shaker R, Lang I. Effect of aging on the deglutitive oral, pharyngeal, and esophageal motor function. [Review]. Dysphagia 1994;9:221.
105. Kahrilas PJ, Dodds WJ, Dent J, et al. Upper esophageal sphincter function during deglutition. Gastroenterology 1988;95:52.
106. Cook IJ, Dodds WJ, Dantas RO, et al. Opening mechanisms of the human upper esophageal sphincter. Am J Phys 1989;257:G748.
107. Cook IJ, Wallace KL, Zagami AS, et al. Mechanisms of pharyngeal dysphagia in lateral medullary syndrome (LMS). Gastroenterology 1996;110:A650.
108. Williams RB, Wallace KL, Ali GN, et al. Biomechanics of failed deglutitive upper esophageal sphincter (UES) relaxation in patients with neurogenic dysphagia. Am J Phys 2002;283:G16.
109. Ali GN, Wallace KL, Laundl TM, et al. Predictors of outcome following cricopharyngeal disruption for pharyngeal dysphagia. Dysphagia 1997;12:133.
110. Mason RJ, Bremner CG, DeMeester TR, et al. Pharyngeal swallowing disorders: selection for and outcome after myotomy. Ann Surg 1998;228:598.
111. Splaingard ML, Hutchins B, Sulton LD, et al. Aspiration in rehabilitation patients: videofluoroscopy vs bedside clinical assessment. Arch Phys Med Rehabil 1988; 69:637.
112. Bath PM, Bath FJ, Smithard DG: Interventions for dysphagia in acute stroke (Cochrane Review), in The Cochrane Library. Oxford:Update Software, 2002. p. CD000323.

113. DePippo KL, Holas MA, Reding MJ, et al. Dysphagia therapy following stroke: a controlled trial. Neurology 1994;44:1655.
114. Baeten C, Hoefnagels J. Feeding via nasogastric tube or percutaneous endoscopic gastrostomy. A comparison. Scand J Gastroenterol 1992;194(Suppl):95.
115. Park RHR, Allison MC, Lang J, et al. Randomised comparison of percutaneous endoscopic gastrostomy and nasogastric tube feeding in patients with persisting neurological dysphagia. BMJ 1992;304:1406.
116. Norton B, Homer WM, Donnelly MT, et al. A randomised prospective comparison of percutaneous endoscopic gastrostomy and nasogastric tube feeding after acute dysphagic stroke. Br Med J 1996;312:13.
117. Dennis MS, Lewis SC, Warlow C, et al. Effect of timing and method of enteral tube feeding for dysphagic stroke patients (FOOD): a multicentre randomised controlled trial [see comment]. Lancet 2005;365:764.
118. St Guily JL, Zhang KX, Perie S, et al. Improvement of dysphagia following cricopharyngeal myotomy in a group of elderly patients. Ann Otol Rhinol Laryngol 1995;104:603.
119. Poirier NC, Bonavina L, Taillefer R, et al. Cricopharyngeal myotomy for neurogenic oropharyngeal dysphagia. J Thorac Cardiovasc Surg 1997;113:233.
120. Taileffer R, Duranceau AC. Manometric and radionuclide assessment of pharyngeal emptying before and after cricopharyngeal myotomy in patients with oculopharyngeal dystrophy. J Thorac Cardiovasc Surg 1988;95:868.
121. Shin T, Tsuda K, Takagi S. Surgical treatment for dysphagia of neuromuscular origin. Folia Phoniatr Logop 1999;51:213.
122. Haapaniemi JJ, Laurikainen EA, Pulkkinen J, et al. Botulinum toxin in the treatment of cricopharyngeal dysphagia. Dysphagia 2001;16:171.

Celiac Disease in the Elderly

Shadi Rashtak, MD[a,b], Joseph A. Murray, MD[a],*

KEYWORDS

• Celiac disease • Elderly • Aging • Gluten malabsorption

Celiac disease is a chronic autoimmune enteropathy occurring in genetically predisposed individuals following ingestion of wheat gluten and related protein fractions of other grains.[1] In patients with celiac disease, tissue transglutaminase binds to gliadin-derived peptides at the gut level and deamidates certain glutamine residues in these peptides. Antigen-presenting cells that express HLA-DQ2 or -DQ8 then present these gliadin-tissue transglutaminase complexes to the T cells. The process of deamidation increases the affinity of the T cells to the gliadin peptides. These T cells then help the B cells to produce antibodies against the gliadin and tissue transglutaminase antigens through epitope spreading. Such inflammatory response results in mucosal damage in forms of lymphocytic infiltration, crypt hyperplasia, and shortening or loss of the villi, which in turn leads to malabsorption.[2–4] As a result, patients present with diarrhea, weight loss, steatorrhea, or malnutrition syndromes such as anemia and diminished bone mass due to deficiencies of important nutrients (iron, folate, calcium, and fat-soluble vitamins).

In addition to the morbidities that result from malabsorption, celiac disease is also associated with other autoimmune diseases and malignancies, leading to higher risk of morbidity and mortality among these patients.[5–7] The risk of autoimmune disorders and cancers particularly increases in older celiac patients and is shown to be associated with the age and the duration of gluten exposure.[8,9]

Despite growing knowledge regarding celiac disease, little is known about this condition in the elderly.[10] This lack of awareness along with the lower frequency of typical symptoms in older celiac patients compared with the younger ones leads to significant delays in the diagnosis of celiac disease in this population, which in turn increases the morbidity and mortality in this group.[5,11] This review focuses on the epidemiology, clinical presentations, complications, diagnosis, and management of celiac disease in the elderly population.

Dr. Joseph Murray is supported by National Institutes of Health grants DK57892, DK71003, and Dr. Shadi Rashtak is supported by the Mayo Foundation.

[a] Division of Gastroenterology and Hepatology, Department of Medicine, Mayo Clinic College of Medicine, 200 First Street, SW, Rochester, MN 55905, USA
[b] Department of Dermatology, Mayo Clinic College of Medicine, 200 First Street, SW, Rochester, MN 55905, USA
* Corresponding author.
E-mail address: murray.joseph@mayo.edu (J.A. Murray).

Gastroenterol Clin N Am 38 (2009) 433–446
doi:10.1016/j.gtc.2009.06.005
0889-8553/09/$ – see front matter © 2009 Elsevier Inc. All rights reserved.

gastro.theclinics.com

EPIDEMIOLOGY

For long time, celiac disease was considered a disease of childhood and was believed to rarely occur in older people.[12] Now there is growing evidence showing an increased rate of diagnosis among adults. Recent reports suggest a trend toward increased incidence of celiac disease, particularly among elderly people.[13] In 1960, only 4% of newly diagnosed celiac disease patients were older than 60 years of age.[14] However, later studies showed that 19% to 34% of new cases of celiac disease are diagnosed in this age group.[11,15–18] A survey of 2440 celiac patients in the United States reported that the proportion of celiac disease patients diagnosed in the elderly is similar to that of those diagnosed before 18 years of age (16% vs 15%, respectively).[10] In accord with these studies, a population-based study of Olmsted County residents in Minnesota reported that celiac disease incidence rates (new cases of celiac disease per 100,000 person-years) in people older than 65 years of age increased significantly from 0.0 in 1950 to 1959 to 15.1 in 2000 to 2001.[13] Our recent data suggest that incidence rates are still increasing among all age groups including the elderly (**Fig. 1**, S. Rashtak, MD, unpublished data, 2009).

The estimated prevalence of celiac disease is now about 1% in the general population.[19,20] In the early 1990s, the prevalence of diagnosed celiac disease in the United States was estimated to be 1 in 5000.[21] Around the same time, reports from Europe showed a 10 to 20 times higher prevalence of celiac disease in Sweden and Italy.[22,23] Later, a large multicenter study in the United States performed serologic screening for celiac disease and found an overall prevalence of 1 in 133 among patients with no risk; a prevalence that was similar to that of European studies.[19] The prevalence of biopsy-proven celiac disease among adults is reported to be 1.2%[20] and a large population-based study on people between 45 and 76 years of age has shown a seropositive prevalence of 1.2% for undetected celiac disease.[24] More recently, a study from

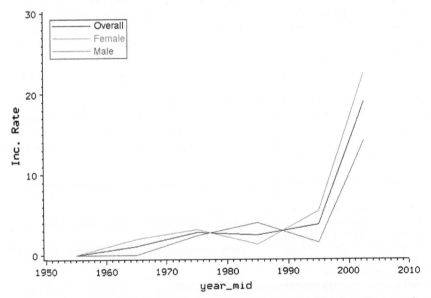

Fig. 1. Increased in the incidence rate of celiac disease in people older than 60 years of age over a 56-year period in Olmsted County, Minnesota (1950–2006). Incidence rate: new cases of CD per 100,000 person-years, adjusted to the United States 2000 white population.

Finland found an even higher prevalence of biopsy-proven celiac disease (2.13%) in older people (52–74 years of age).[25] A recent study has demonstrated that celiac disease may truly occur for the first time in an elderly individual, despite a lifelong apparent tolerance of gluten ingestion, not merely be diagnosed at this age.[26]

Similar to other autoimmune disorders, celiac disease occurs more frequently in women, with a female to male ratio of 2:1.[10,27] In both men and women the incidence rate of celiac disease continues to increase until 65 years of age, at which point the incidence rate begins to decrease in women whereas it continues to increase gradually in men. Nonetheless, the incidence rate still remains higher in women older than 65 years of age compared with men of the same age.[13,15]

CLINICAL PRESENTATION

It has become apparent over the last 20 years that celiac disease produces a spectrum of clinical features that extend from severe malabsorption with profound nutritional deficiencies to presentation with a single symptom such as anemia, accelerated osteoporosis, or osteomalacia. For unknown reasons, presentation of intestinal symptoms is less prominent in elderly celiac patients compared with younger ones.[28] Instead, the signs of micronutrient deficiencies may be the first and often the only presentation of the disease in the elderly.

Anemia is present in 60% to 80% of elderly patients with celiac disease[11,17] and has been mainly attributed to the deficiency of micronutrients, particularly iron. Deficiencies of other nutrients such as folate and vitamin B12 may account for a smaller percentage of anemia in these patients which, in conjunction with iron deficiency, sometimes causes dimorphic peripheral smear.[28–32] It is hypothesized that anemia of celiac disease is multifactorial, and systemic inflammation may also be a contributing factor in the etiology of anemia in celiac disease.[29] It has been shown that some anemic celiac patients have high levels of ferritin (an acute phase reactant) and erythrocyte sedimentation rate, suggestive of systemic inflammation and anemia of chronic disease in these patients.[29,33]

Although abdominal symptoms are still common in elderly celiac patients, many of these individuals present with milder symptoms such as abdominal bloating, flatulence, and abdominal discomfort, which make the diagnosis more difficult. The classic malabsorptive symptoms such as diarrhea, weight loss, and abdominal pain are less common in elderly celiac patients.[34] It should be noted, though, that celiac disease is the most common cause of steatorrhea in people older than 50 years of age and the second most common cause in those older than 65 years.[35] Nonetheless, it seems that malabsorptive-induced bowel dysfunction is tolerated well among elderly people. Diarrhea, although a common feature, may be mild or intermittent in older celiac patients and a few patients may even present with constipation.[17,36] In addition, some patients may not present with any intestinal symptoms at all, a condition called silent celiac disease.[37]

Deficiencies of calcium and vitamin D may be another clinical feature of celiac disease leading to decreased bone mass, particularly in elderly patients who are already susceptible to metabolic bone disorders.[38,39] Malnutrition can also cause hypoalbuminemia in these patients, which additionally may lead to hypocalcemia and hypomagnesemia. Hypoalbuminemia itself can also present with edema and ascites in these patients.[17] In about 20% of celiac patients, hepatocellular changes may occur, presenting with an abnormal liver function test, a condition called celiac hepatitis. This condition in turn can lead to further investigation for exclusion of other causes of the liver disease.[40] It has been shown that a gluten-free diet has beneficial effects on resolution of symptoms in celiac hepatitis.[41]

In addition to the gastrointestinal symptoms and malnutrition disorders that result from intestinal involvement, celiac disease may also present through its associated disorders and complications. Dermatitis herpetiformis, well recognized as the skin manifestation of celiac disease, may be the first presentation of gluten sensitivity in celiac patients.[42] Dermatitis herpetiformis occurs in about 25% of patients with celiac disease and is more common in men than women, with a male to female ratio of about 2:1.[43,44] The average age of presentation is about 40 years, with most patients aged between 20 and 70 years. Nonetheless it can occur at any age, even in childhood. The disease presents with extremely pruritic papulovesicular rash on the extensor surfaces (elbows, knees, buttocks, and scalp).[44,45] About 80% of dermatitis herpetiformis patients show intestinal alterations consistent with celiac disease in the endoscopic or histopathologic evaluation. However, only 20% of these patients initially have gastrointestinal symptoms of celiac disease.[46] The diagnosis is made by direct immunofluorescence staining of a perilesional skin specimen showing granular IgA deposition in the dermoepidermal junction, more prominently within the papillary tips.[45] The basis of therapy relies on instruction of a gluten-free diet, which controls the underlying pathology and results in slow resolution of symptoms. Dapsone therapy could be used for suppression of initial symptoms and even intermittently for occasional outbreaks.[45]

Other autoimmune diseases are also frequently associated with celiac disease and may provide clues for suspicion of celiac disease in an elderly patient. Autoimmune thyroid disorders are the most common associated autoimmune diseases in elderly celiac patients, with most patients presenting with hypothyroidism.[28,47] In addition, the risk of intestinal lymphoma and other celiac disease-associated malignancies is higher in elderly people[48] and some patients may present with acute complications of such diseases, including intestinal obstruction or perforation.[49–51] On occasion celiac disease may present with cavitation of mesenteric lymph nodes and splenic atrophy, or with intestinal ulceration with or without underlying malignancy.[52–54]

DIAGNOSIS

Clinical diagnosis of celiac disease in the elderly can be challenging for primary care physicians, which may be in part due to the subtle clinical symptoms, low index of suspicion for celiac disease in elderly people, and distraction toward more threatening conditions such as malignancies.[10,28] For example, the mild changes in bowel habits may be easily attributed to the functional changes in the intestinal tract due to diseases such as irritable bowel syndrome, mood disorders (anxiety, depression, and so forth), or even be considered as part of the normal aging process. A survey of elderly celiac patients has shown that a substantial number of these patients are incorrectly diagnosed as irritable bowel syndrome many years before their celiac disease is diagnosed, leading to an average delay of 17 years in the diagnosis.[10] In addition, symptoms such as anemia in an elderly celiac patient may lead to extensive evaluation to rule out colon cancer before celiac disease is even considered.

Several diseases are considered in an elderly patient who presents with symptoms of malabsorption. Small intestine bacterial overgrowth, small bowel ischemia, and exocrine pancreatic insufficiency (in association with chronic pancreatitis or pancreatic cancer) may be more common in the elderly and sometimes can manifest with chronic malabsorption. These disorders can mimic celiac disease in an older patient or can occur in elderly celiac patients due to their advanced age.[37,55] Autoimmune enteropathy, albeit an extremely rare condition, has also been described in older patients. Nongranulomatous enterocolitis or self-limited enteritis may be seen in elderly patients too. Malignancies, in particular cancers of the gastrointestinal tract, should be listed as part of the differential diagnosis in an elderly patient presenting with anemia or weight loss.

In general, elderly celiac patients are probably just as likely to have serologic abnormalities as younger patients, and the HLA association with celiac disease persists in this age group. The diagnosis for celiac disease in elderly patients proceeds along the same lines as in younger celiac patients. Serologic tests are frequently used for the diagnosis and follow-up of celiac disease. The basis of serologic testing for celiac disease relies on the measurement of (auto)antibodies, particularly the IgA isotype. The diagnosis is usually confirmed by histologic evaluation of small intestinal biopsy, which is the gold standard test for celiac disease diagnosis. It is important for the primary care physicians to be aware of the advantages and disadvantages of each diagnostic test and select the best option based on each patient's individual needs.

The current available serologic tests for celiac disease diagnosis include antiendomysial (EMA) and antitissue transglutaminase (TTG) autoantibodies as well as antibodies against gliadin peptides (**Table 1**). For EMA testing, monkey esophagus or human umbilical cord is used as a substrate. The test is considered highly specific, with a reported specificity of close to 100% in most studies.[56,57] The sensitivity is also high (>90%) in most reports; however, recent studies have shown that the sensitivity decreases significantly in patients with milder degree of intestinal damage and can reach as low as 30% in patients with partial villous atrophy.[56–58] The cost of EMA testing is high, which in addition to the subjective and qualitative nature of the test, limits its applicability for routine diagnosis of celiac disease. The TTG IgA test, on the other hand, does not have these limitations of EMA testing, and has a comparable sensitivity (~90%) and specificity (~95%) to that of EMA.[59] TTG IgA measurement is therefore recommended as the initial screening test for celiac disease.[1] Antigliadin antibodies that were once used frequently for celiac disease diagnosis are no longer recommended due to their poor sensitivity and specificity.[59] Instead, a newly developed assay that uses deamidated gliadin peptides (DGP) as the antigen has been shown to be significantly more accurate than the conventional gliadin antibody testing for celiac disease diagnosis.[60,61]

Table 1
Estimated range of sensitivity and specificity for serologic diagnosis of celiac disease based on reports from studies in adult population (the outlier results of some studies are excluded)

Test	Sensitivity (%)	Specificity (%)
EMA IgA[59]	85–100	~100
TTG IgA[56,59]	80–100	90–100
TTG IgG[56,60]	20–60	>95
DGP IgA[60,61]	75–95	>95
DGP IgG[60–62]	65–90	>95
Gliadin IgA[56,59]	60–90	80–100
Gliadin IgG[56,59,60]	40–80	70–90

Abbreviations: DGP, deamidated gliadin peptides; EMA, endomysial antibody; TTG, tissue transglutaminase.

Despite good sensitivity and specificity of these antibody tests, several celiac patients may be missed on the basis of serologic testing alone. Similar to EMA testing, TTG and DGP antibodies have more false-negative results in patients with a milder degree of enteropathy.[60,62] Another possibility for a false-negative test in a celiac patient is IgA deficiency. In this setting, IgG isotype of relevant antibodies can be used as a diagnostic test. It has been shown that DGP IgG is significantly more sensitive than TTG IgG for celiac disease diagnosis and therefore may be more helpful in these circumstances.[60,62] The recently developed multiplex immunoassay can simultaneously measure TTG and DGP IgA and IgG antibodies with a similar accuracy to that of the enzyme-linked immunosorbent assay.[62] Combination testing may increase the sensitivity and detection of IgA-deficient patients, but still a number of celiac patients, particularly those with partial villous atrophy, remain seronegative for all of the relevant antibodies. It is therefore important that patients undergo intestinal biopsy when there is a high suspicion for celiac disease despite a negative serology.[60,63] Intestinal biopsy can also confirm the diagnosis in seropositive patients and provide baseline information regarding the degree of intestinal damage for further evaluation of response to the treatment.

The histologic diagnosis of celiac disease is made by the presence of enteropathy in the duodenal biopsy specimens. Increased intraepithelial lymphocyte infiltrate, crypt hyperplasia, and villous atrophy are the three histologic features of celiac enteropathy.[64] There are no age-related changes in the intestine of older individuals and therefore the histologic diagnosis of celiac disease does not differ from that of young patients.[37] Although one might hesitate to subject a very elderly patient with multiple comorbidities to intestinal biopsy as a primary or initial test for celiac disease, older patients are more likely to undergo endoscopy (to exclude other causes of their symptoms) and to have their first diagnosis made by duodenal biopsies rather than serology. It would be important in these patients to provide supportive evidence by means of specific serologic testing and, if negative, compatible HLA genetic susceptibility for celiac disease.[60,62,63] Close follow-up of elderly patients is important to ensure appropriate response and the correction of symptoms, and consequences of malabsorption. It should be noted that healing of the intestine may be slow in older patients diagnosed with celiac disease.

COMPLICATIONS
Autoimmune Disorders

Celiac disease has many features of an autoimmune disorder, including strong association with major histocompatibility complex (MHC) class II molecules, presence of (antitissue transglutaminase) autoantibodies, multiorgan involvement, and dysregulation of innate and adaptive immune responses.[65–69] One of the autoimmune features of celiac disease is its common occurrence with other autoimmune disorders.[67,68] It is important that physicians be aware of these associations, as it can particularly improve case finding among elderly patients with less typical symptoms. Moreover, knowing the increased risk of such diseases in celiac patients leads to better management in terms of diagnosis and treatment of the associated autoimmune disorder.

In general, autoimmune disorders are 3 to 10 times more prevalent in celiac patients and 5 times more prevalent in family members of celiac patients compared with the general population.[70–74] Similarly, celiac disease occurs more frequently in patients with autoimmune disorders[75–77] as well as in those who have a relative affected with celiac disease.[19] The risk is much higher when both conditions are present together. About 25% of the individuals who have both an autoimmune disorder and a positive family history of celiac disease are found to have celiac enteropathy through screening.[74] It has been shown that the risk of autoimmunity is directly associated with age at the diagnosis of celiac disease.[8,78] Although some investigators attribute this association to the duration of gluten exposure,[8] others have found only age as a significant predictor of autoimmunity in the adult population.[78]

The association of celiac disease with autoimmune diseases such as type 1 diabetes and autoimmune thyroid disorders (Hashimoto thyroiditis and Graves disease) is well established.[79–84] In contrast to children, in whom type 1 diabetes is more commonly associated with celiac disease,[80,81] older celiac patients present with lower prevalence of type 1 diabetes. Instead, autoimmune thyroid disorders are frequently associated with celiac disease in the elderly.[82,85]

Involvement of hepatobiliary and nervous systems in celiac disease also occurs through immune-mediated processes. Autoimmune cholestatic liver disorders such as autoimmune hepatitis, primary biliary cirrhosis, and primary sclerosing cholangitis are more frequent in celiac patients than in the general population.[41,86] These disorders are different from celiac hepatitis, which does not occur through autoimmune processes. The response to the dietary treatment is also different between autoimmune liver diseases and celiac hepatitis. In contrast to celiac hepatitis that has a good response to a gluten-free diet, autoimmune cholestatic liver damage does not seem to respond efficiently to gluten exclusion.[41,86]

Ataxia and neuropathy are two main neurologic complications of celiac disease that can particularly be problematic in elderly patients.[87–89] The disturbance of balance control due to involvement of the nervous system leads to a higher risk of falls in these patients, which further increases the risk of bone fractures, particularly in elderly celiac patients with low bone density. Cognitive impairment, in particular accelerated dementia, has also been seen in older patients with celiac disease and unfortunately may not respond to a gluten-free diet.[90]

Refractory Celiac Disease

Refractory celiac disease (RCD) is defined as significant malabsorption in a patient with severe enteropathy who has had a lack of initial response to a gluten-free diet or recurrence of symptoms despite strict adherence to the diet. RCD is a diagnosis of exclusion. The most common cause of unresponsiveness in celiac disease is gluten contamination of the diet.[91] Even minute amounts of gluten used in pills, capsules, envelope adhesive, modified food starch, preservatives, and stabilizers can prevent healing of the intestine, resulting in the persistence of symptoms. Other conditions that should be ruled out before the diagnosis of RCD is made include microscopic colitis, pancreatic insufficiency, small bacterial overgrowth, irritable bowel syndrome, and lactose intolerance.[91,92] There are rare enteropathies that can mimic celiac disease pathology in the elderly and may cause apparent failure of response to treatment. These include self-limited enteritis, autoimmune enteropathy, collagenous sprue, and even nonsteroidal anti-inflammatory drug injury.[93,94]

RCD is categorized into two types based on the immunophenotype of intraepithelial lymphocytes: polyclonal with normal phenotype in RCD I and monoclonal with abnormal phenotype in RCD II.[95,96] About 5% of celiac patients may develop RCD, with most patients belonging to the elderly group. In a study of 57 Mayo Clinic patients, the median (range) of age for RCD diagnosis was 58 (30–76) and 70 (47–76) years for RCD I and RCD II, respectively.[97] The diagnosis of celiac disease in half of the RCD patients was made after 54 (in RCD I) and 61 (in RCD II) years of age. In the same study, the cumulative 5-year survival was reported to be 80% in RCD I but just 45% in RCD II patients, and the main causes of death were refractory state (in RCD I) and enteropathy-associated T-cell lymphoma (in RCD II).[97] In those RCD II patients who develop enteropathy-associated lymphoma, the prognosis is poor.[98] In the new system proposed for the staging of RCD, age (older than 65 years) was found to be one of the five prognostic factors with a negative effect on the survival of RCD patients.[97]

Malignancy

The risk of malignancy is increased in celiac patients, particularly in those with advanced age. The relative risk for the development of intestinal lymphoma in celiac patients is reported to be 5 to 300 in different studies.[99,100] The incidence of lymphoma is much greater after the sixth decade of life, and it occurs more commonly in patients who were diagnosed with celiac disease between 50 and 80 years of age.[9] Enteropathy-associated T-cell lymphomas have the strongest association with celiac disease and present with multifocal and ulcerative lesions. This association explains the high rate of bowel perforation in these patients, which may sometimes be the initial presentation of the disease. There is also a high risk of perforation on commencement of chemotherapy. Non-Hodgkin lymphomas and adenocarcinomas of the gastrointestinal tract are also more common in celiac patients than expected.[48,101] The risk of breast cancer is reduced in celiac patients.[6,102] Most studies show an increased mortality rate in celiac patients, which has not always been attributed to the increased cancer risk in these patients.[6,7,103] Even asymptomatic patients (silent celiac disease) have a higher mortality rate compared with the general population.[104] A gluten-free diet has been shown to have a protective effect on the risk of malignancy in celiac patients.[101,105]

MANAGEMENT

The treatment of celiac disease relies on the basis of strict adherence to a gluten-free diet. Despite a high rate of dietary compliance reported in elderly celiac patients,[11] the management of celiac disease in these patients has some specific challenges. First, patients usually have a lifetime of dietary habits that may be hard to break. They may also have limited financial or social resources and limited mobility, restricting their ability to travel to gluten-free suppliers. Elderly patients may be residing in assisted living facilities where it may be difficult to provide them with a gluten-free diet. Additional issues relate to poor nutritional intake, and impaired vision limiting their ability to read ingredient lists that are often minute in size.

Patients should be encouraged to seek out community support, and family members should be recruited and probably should participate in the patient's dietary consultation. Direct communication between the dietician and the director of food services at the patient's institution, if institutionalized, are likely necessary to achieve a gluten-free diet. In the very elderly or debilitated patient who has minor symptoms, consideration of not treating the patient with a gluten-free diet may have some rationale. However, it should be noted that patients can often have a dramatic improvement in chronic symptoms, even nongastrointestinal symptoms, after adherence to a gluten-free diet, and the opportunity for this recovery should not be lost.

Patients diagnosed with celiac disease should be referred to a gastroenterologist to ensure optimum management of the disease and its associate complications.[36] It is important that patients be investigated for the presence of anemia, calcium and vitamin D deficiency, osteoporosis, and thyroid and liver diseases during the follow-up visits. Calcium and vitamin supplementation should be encouraged in these patients and should be used in conjunction with bisphosphonates if osteoporosis is present.

SUMMARY

Celiac disease is a common disorder not only in the young but also in the elderly. Celiac disease may linger for many years before the diagnosis, causing subtle or troubling symptoms, and may present for the first time with serious fatal complications. A greater awareness of the incidence and clinical presentation of celiac disease in the elderly is essential to prevent long delays in the diagnosis. Although the treatment of celiac disease is straightforward, the elderly present specific challenges in the management of their celiac disease, particularly in view of making radical changes to diet as well as coping with the complications of longstanding malabsorption. A comprehensive, multidisciplinary approach to the management of celiac disease should result in reduced morbidity in these patients. A management approach tailored to the particular challenges presented by elderly celiac patients is crucial to their success.

REFERENCES

1. Green PH, Cellier C. Celiac disease. N Engl J Med 2007;357(17):1731–43.
2. Guandalini S, Gokhale R. Update on immunologic basis of celiac disease. Curr Opin Gastroenterol 2002;18(1):95–100.
3. Marietta EV, Rashtak S, Murray JA. Correlation analysis of celiac sprue tissue transglutaminase and deamidated gliadin IgG/IgA. World J Gastroenterol 2009;15(7):845–8.
4. Sollid LM, Molberg O, McAdam S, et al. Autoantibodies in coeliac disease: tissue transglutaminase–guilt by association? Gut 1997;41(6):851–2.
5. Hovdenak N. [Celiac disease in the elderly]. Tidsskr Nor Laegeforen 1995; 115(12):1491–3 [Norwegian].
6. West J, Logan RF, Smith CJ, et al. Malignancy and mortality in people with coeliac disease: population based cohort study. BMJ 2004;329(7468):716–9.
7. Viljamaa M, Kaukinen K, Pukkala E, et al. Malignancies and mortality in patients with coeliac disease and dermatitis herpetiformis: 30-year population-based study. Dig Liver Dis 2006;38(6):374–80.
8. Ventura A, Magazzu G, Greco L. Duration of exposure to gluten and risk for autoimmune disorders in patients with celiac disease. SIGEP Study Group for Autoimmune Disorders in Celiac Disease. Gastroenterology 1999;117(2):297–303.
9. Cooper BT, Holmes GK, Cooke WT. Lymphoma risk in coeliac disease of later life. Digestion 1982;23(2):89–92.
10. Patel D, Kalkat P, Baisch D, et al. Celiac disease in the elderly. Gerontology 2005;51(3):213–4.
11. Hankey GL, Holmes GK. Coeliac disease in the elderly. Gut 1994;35(1):65–7.
12. Coeliac disease in the elderly. Lancet 1984;1(8380):775–6.
13. Murray JA, Van Dyke C, Plevak MF, et al. Trends in the identification and clinical features of celiac disease in a North American community, 1950–2001. Clin Gastroenterol Hepatol 2003;1(1):19–27.
14. Green PA, Wollaeger EE. The clinical behavior of sprue in the United States. Gastroenterology 1960;38:399–38418.
15. Swinson CM, Levi AJ. Is coeliac disease underdiagnosed? Br Med J 1980; 281(6250):1258–60.

16. Campbell CB, Roberts RK, Cowen AE. The changing clinical presentation of coeliac disease in adults. Med J Aust 1977;1(4):89–93.

17. Freeman H. Clinical spectrum of biopsy-defined celiac disease in the elderly. Can J Gastroenterol 1995;9(1):42–6.

18. Beaumont DM, Mian MS. Coeliac disease in old age: 'a catch in the rye'. Age Ageing 1998;27(4):535–8.

19. Fasano A, Berti I, Gerarduzzi T, et al. Prevalence of celiac disease in at-risk and not-at-risk groups in the United States: a large multicenter study. Arch Intern Med 2003;163(3):286–92.

20. Cook HB, Burt MJ, Collett JA, et al. Adult coeliac disease: prevalence and clinical significance. J Gastroenterol Hepatol 2000;15(9):1032–6.

21. Talley NJ, Valdovinos M, Petterson TM, et al. Epidemiology of celiac sprue: a community-based study. Am J Gastroenterol 1994;89(6):843–6.

22. Ascher H, Kristiansson B. The highest incidence of celiac disease in Europe: the Swedish experience. J Pediatr Gastroenterol Nutr 1997;24(5):S3–6.

23. Catassi C, Fabiani E, Ratsch IM, et al. Celiac disease in the general population: should we treat asymptomatic cases? J Pediatr Gastroenterol Nutr 1997;24(5): S10–2 [discussion: S2–3].

24. West J, Logan RF, Hill PG, et al. Seroprevalence, correlates, and characteristics of undetected coeliac disease in England. Gut 2003;52(7):960–5.

25. Vilppula A, Collin P, Maki M, et al. Undetected coeliac disease in the elderly: a biopsy-proven population-based study. Dig Liver Dis 2008;40(10):809–13.

26. Lohi S, Mustalahti K, Kaukinen K, et al. Increasing prevalence of coeliac disease over time. Aliment Pharmacol Ther 2007;26(9):1217–25.

27. Feighery C, Weir DG, Whelan A, et al. Diagnosis of gluten-sensitive enteropathy: is exclusive reliance on histology appropriate? Eur J Gastroenterol Hepatol 1998;10(11):919–25.

28. Freeman HJ. Adult celiac disease in the elderly. World J Gastroenterol 2008; 14(45):6911–4.

29. Harper JW, Holleran SF, Ramakrishnan R, et al. Anemia in celiac disease is multifactorial in etiology. Am J Hematol 2007;82(11):996–1000.

30. Bode S, Gudmand-Hoyer E. Symptoms and haematologic features in consecutive adult coeliac patients. Scand J Gastroenterol 1996;31(1):54–60.

31. Pittschieler K. [Folic acid concentration in the serum and erythrocytes of patients with celiac disease]. Padiatr Padol 1986;21(4):363–6 [German].

32. Dahele A, Ghosh S. Vitamin B12 deficiency in untreated celiac disease. Am J Gastroenterol 2001;96(3):745–50.

33. Gariballa S, Forster S. Effects of acute-phase response on nutritional status and clinical outcome of hospitalized patients. Nutrition 2006;22(7–8):750–7.

34. Cranney A, Zarkadas M, Graham ID, et al. The Canadian celiac health survey. Dig Dis Sci 2007;52(4):1087–95.

35. Price HL, Gazzard BG, Dawson AM. Steatorrhoea in the elderly. Br Med J 1977; 1(6076):1582–4.

36. Johnson MW, Ellis HJ, Asante MA, et al. Celiac disease in the elderly. Nat Clin Pract Gastroenterol Hepatol 2008;5(12):697–706.

37. Holt PR. Intestinal malabsorption in the elderly. Dig Dis 2007;25(2):144–50.

38. Gallagher JC, Riggs BL, Eisman J, et al. Intestinal calcium absorption and serum vitamin D metabolites in normal subjects and osteoporotic patients: effect of age and dietary calcium. J Clin Invest 1979;64(3):729–36.

39. Bullamore JR, Wilkinson R, Gallagher JC, et al. Effect of age on calcium absorption. Lancet 1970;2(7672):535–7.

40. Freeman H, Lemoyne M, Pare P. Coeliac disease. Best Pract Res Clin Gastroenterol 2002;16(1):37–49.
41. Rubio-Tapia A, Murray JA. Liver involvement in celiac disease. Minerva Medicoleg 2008;99(6):595–604.
42. Reunala T. Dermatitis herpetiformis: coeliac disease of the skin. Annu Mediaev 1998;30(5):416–8.
43. Collin P, Reunala T. Recognition and management of the cutaneous manifestations of celiac disease: a guide for dermatologists. Am J Clin Dermatol 2003;4(1):13–20.
44. Gawkrodger DJ, Blackwell JN, Gilmour HM, et al. Dermatitis herpetiformis: diagnosis, diet and demography. Gut 1984;25(2):151–7.
45. Nicolas ME, Krause PK, Gibson LE, et al. Dermatitis herpetiformis. Int J Dermatol 2003;42(8):588–600.
46. Gregory B, Ho VC. Cutaneous manifestations of gastrointestinal disorders. Part II. J Am Acad Dermatol 1992;26(3 Pt 2):371–83.
47. Midhagen G, Jarnerot G, Kraaz W. Adult coeliac disease within a defined geographic area in Sweden. A study of prevalence and associated diseases. Scand J Gastroenterol 1988;23(8):1000–4.
48. Swinson CM, Slavin G, Coles EC, et al. Coeliac disease and malignancy. Lancet 1983;1(8316):111–5.
49. Johnston SD, Watson RG. Small bowel lymphoma in unrecognized coeliac disease: a cause for concern? Eur J Gastroenterol Hepatol 2000;12(6):645–8.
50. Connon JJ, McFarland J, Kelly A, et al. Acute abdominal complications of coeliac disease. Scand J Gastroenterol 1975;10(8):843–6.
51. Finan PJ, Thompson MR. Surgical presentation of small bowel lymphoma in adult coeliac disease. Postgrad Med J 1980;56(662):859–61.
52. Matuchansky C, Colin R, Hemet J, et al. Cavitation of mesenteric lymph nodes, splenic atrophy, and a flat small intestinal mucosa. Report of six cases. Gastroenterology 1984;87(3):606–14.
53. Tonder M, Sorlie D, Kearney MS. Adult coeliac disease. A case with ulceration, dermatitis herpetiformis and reticulosarcoma. Scand J Gastroenterol 1976; 11(1):107–11.
54. Robertson DA, Dixon MF, Scott BB, et al. Small intestinal ulceration: diagnostic difficulties in relation to coeliac disease. Gut 1983;24(6):565–74.
55. Rubio-Tapia A, Barton SH, Rosenblatt JE, et al. Prevalence of small intestine bacterial overgrowth diagnosed by quantitative culture of intestinal aspirate in celiac disease. J Clin Gastroenterol 2009;43(2):157–61.
56. Rostom A, Dube C, Cranney A, et al. The diagnostic accuracy of serologic tests for celiac disease: a systematic review. Gastroenterology 2005;128(4 Suppl 1): S38–46.
57. Rostami K, Kerckhaert J, Tiemessen R, et al. Sensitivity of antiendomysium and antigliadin antibodies in untreated celiac disease: disappointing in clinical practice. Am J Gastroenterol 1999;94(4):888–94.
58. Rostami K, Kerckhaert J, von Blomberg BM, et al. SAT and serology in adult coeliacs, seronegative coeliac disease seems a reality. Neth J Med 1998; 53(1):15–9.
59. Hill ID. What are the sensitivity and specificity of serologic tests for celiac disease? Do sensitivity and specificity vary in different populations? Gastroenterology 2005;128(4 Suppl 1):S25–32.
60. Rashtak S, Ettore MW, Homburger HA, et al. Comparative usefulness of deamidated gliadin antibodies in the diagnosis of celiac disease. Clin Gastroenterol Hepatol 2008;6(4):426–32, quiz 370.

61. Sugai E, Vazquez H, Nachman F, et al. Accuracy of testing for antibodies to synthetic gliadin-related peptides in celiac disease. Clin Gastroenterol Hepatol 2006;4(9):1112–7.
62. Rashtak S, Ettore MW, Homburger HA, et al. Combination testing for antibodies in the diagnosis of coeliac disease: comparison of multiplex immunoassay and ELISA methods. Aliment Pharmacol Ther 2008;28(6):805–13.
63. Rashtak S, Murray JA. Tailored testing for celiac disease. Ann Intern Med 2007; 147(5):339–41.
64. Marsh MN. Gluten, major histocompatibility complex, and the small intestine. A molecular and immunobiologic approach to the spectrum of gluten sensitivity ('celiac sprue'). Gastroenterology 1992;102(1):330–54.
65. Sollid LM, Thorsby E. HLA susceptibility genes in celiac disease: genetic mapping and role in pathogenesis. Gastroenterology 1993;105(3):910–22.
66. Spurkland A, Sollid LM, Polanco I, et al. HLA-DR and -DQ genotypes of celiac disease patients serologically typed to be non-DR3 or non-DR5/7. Hum Immunol 1992;35(3):188–92.
67. Rubio-Tapia A, Murray JA. Celiac disease beyond the gut. Clin Gastroenterol Hepatol 2008;6(7):722–3.
68. Sollid LM, Jabri B. Is celiac disease an autoimmune disorder? Curr Opin Immunol 2005;17(6):595–600.
69. Briani C, Samaroo D, Alaedini A. Celiac disease: from gluten to autoimmunity. Autoimmun Rev 2008;7(8):644–50.
70. Volta U, De Franceschi L, Molinaro N, et al. Organ-specific autoantibodies in coeliac disease: do they represent an epiphenomenon or the expression of associated autoimmune disorders? Ital J Gastroenterol Hepatol 1997;29(1):18–21.
71. Hernandez L, Green PH. Extraintestinal manifestations of celiac disease. Curr Gastroenterol Rep 2006;8(5):383–9.
72. Cosnes J, Cellier C, Viola S, et al. Incidence of autoimmune diseases in celiac disease: protective effect of the gluten-free diet. Clin Gastroenterol Hepatol 2008;6(7):753–8.
73. Cataldo F, Marino V. Increased prevalence of autoimmune diseases in first-degree relatives of patients with celiac disease. J Pediatr Gastroenterol Nutr 2003;36(4):470–3.
74. Petaros P, Martelossi S, Tommasini A, et al. Prevalence of autoimmune disorders in relatives of patients with celiac disease. Dig Dis Sci 2002;47(7):1427–31.
75. Fasano A. Systemic autoimmune disorders in celiac disease. Curr Opin Gastroenterol 2006;22(6):674–9.
76. Ch'ng CL, Jones MK, Kingham JG. Celiac disease and autoimmune thyroid disease. Clin Med Res 2007;5(3):184–92.
77. Murray JA. Celiac disease in patients with an affected member, type 1 diabetes, iron-deficiency, or osteoporosis? Gastroenterology 2005;128(4 Suppl 1):S52–6.
78. Sategna Guidetti C, Solerio E, Scaglione N, et al. Duration of gluten exposure in adult coeliac disease does not correlate with the risk for autoimmune disorders. Gut 2001;49(4):502–5.
79. Talal AH, Murray JA, Goeken JA, et al. Celiac disease in an adult population with insulin-dependent diabetes mellitus: use of endomysial antibody testing. Am J Gastroenterol 1997;92(8):1280–4.
80. Salardi S, Volta U, Zucchini S, et al. Prevalence of celiac disease in children with type 1 diabetes mellitus increased in the mid-1990 s: an 18-year longitudinal study based on anti-endomysial antibodies. J Pediatr Gastroenterol Nutr 2008; 46(5):612–4.

81. Ludvigsson JF, Ludvigsson J, Ekbom A, et al. Celiac disease and risk of subsequent type 1 diabetes: a general population cohort study of children and adolescents. Diabetes Care 2006;29(11):2483–8.

82. Sategna-Guidetti C, Bruno M, Mazza E, et al. Autoimmune thyroid diseases and coeliac disease. Eur J Gastroenterol Hepatol 1998;10(11):927–31.

83. Counsell CE, Ruddell WS. Association between coeliac disease and autoimmune thyroid disease. Gut 1995;36(3):475–6.

84. Ansaldi N, Palmas T, Corrias A, et al. Autoimmune thyroid disease and celiac disease in children. J Pediatr Gastroenterol Nutr 2003;37(1):63–6.

85. Collin P, Reunala T, Pukkala E, et al. Coeliac disease–associated disorders and survival. Gut 1994;35(9):1215–8.

86. Volta U, Rodrigo L, Granito A, et al. Celiac disease in autoimmune cholestatic liver disorders. Am J Gastroenterol 2002;97(10):2609–13.

87. Green PH, Alaedini A, Sander HW, et al. Mechanisms underlying celiac disease and its neurologic manifestations. Cell Mol Life Sci 2005;62(7–8):791–9.

88. Bushara KO. Neurologic presentation of celiac disease. Gastroenterology 2005; 128(4 Suppl 1):S92–7.

89. Briani C, Zara G, Alaedini A, et al. Neurological complications of celiac disease and autoimmune mechanisms: a prospective study. J Neuroimmunol 2008; 195(1–2):171–5.

90. Hu WT, Murray JA, Greenaway MC, et al. Cognitive impairment and celiac disease. Arch Neurol 2006;63(10):1440–6.

91. Abdulkarim AS, Burgart LJ, See J, et al. Etiology of nonresponsive celiac disease: results of a systematic approach. Am J Gastroenterol 2002;97(8): 2016–21.

92. Leffler DA, Dennis M, Hyett B, et al. Etiologies and predictors of diagnosis in nonresponsive celiac disease. Clin Gastroenterol Hepatol 2007;5(4):445–50.

93. Goldstein NS. Non-gluten sensitivity-related small bowel villous flattening with increased intraepithelial lymphocytes: not all that flattens is celiac sprue. Am J Clin Pathol 2004;121(4):546–50.

94. Akram S, Murray JA, Pardi DS, et al. Adult autoimmune enteropathy: Mayo Clinic Rochester experience. Clin Gastroenterol Hepatol 2007;5(11):1282–90, qu 45.

95. Cellier C, Delabesse E, Helmer C, et al. Refractory sprue, coeliac disease, and enteropathy-associated T-cell lymphoma. French Coeliac Disease Study Group. Lancet 2000;356(9225):203–8.

96. Patey-Mariaud De Serre N, Cellier C, Jabri B, et al. Distinction between coeliac disease and refractory sprue: a simple immunohistochemical method. Histopathology 2000;37(1):70–7.

97. Rubio-Tapia A, Kelly DG, Lahr BD, et al. Clinical staging and survival in refractory celiac disease: a single center experience. Gastroenterology 2009;136(1): 99–107, quiz 352–3.

98. Al-Toma A, Verbeek WH, Hadithi M, et al. Survival in refractory coeliac disease and enteropathy-associated T-cell lymphoma: retrospective evaluation of single-centre experience. Gut 2007;56(10):1373–8.

99. Goddard CJ, Gillett HR. Complications of coeliac disease: are all patients at risk? Postgrad Med J 2006;82(973):705–12.

100. Green PHR, Stavropoulos SN, Panagi SG, et al. Characteristics of adult celiac disease in the USA: results of a national survey. Am J Gastroenterol 2001; 96(1):126–31.

101. Holmes GK, Prior P, Lane MR, et al. Malignancy in coeliac disease—effect of a gluten free diet. Gut 1989;30(3):333–8.

102. Brottveit M, Lundin KE. [Cancer risk in coeliac disease]. Tidsskr Nor Laegeforen 2008;128(20):2312–5 [Norwegian].
103. Anderson LA, McMillan SA, Watson RG, et al. Malignancy and mortality in a population-based cohort of patients with coeliac disease or "gluten sensitivity". World J Gastroenterol 2007;13(1):146–51.
104. Rubio-Tapia A, Kyle RA, Kaplan EL, et al. Increased prevalence and mortality in undiagnosed celiac disease. Gastroenterology 2009.
105. Silano M, Volta U, Vincenzi AD, et al. Effect of a gluten-free diet on the risk of enteropathy-associated T-cell lymphoma in celiac disease. Dig Dis Sci 2008; 53(4):972–6.

Inflammatory Bowel Disease in the Elderly

Michael F. Picco, MD, PhD*, John R. Cangemi, MD

KEYWORDS

- Inflammatory bowel disease • Elderly
- Geriatric • Colitis • Crohn

Much has been learned about the natural history, prognosis, and treatment of inflammatory bowel disease (IBD) in the elderly since this topic was last reviewed in *Gastroenterology Clinics of North America*.[1] Recent studies have suggested important differences between older and younger patients in the presentation and prognosis of Crohn disease (CD) and ulcerative colitis (UC), yet many questions remain unanswered. Whereas as the population ages the definition of "elderly" may change, the proportion of older patients with IBD will increase with time. The understanding of features of these diseases and other disorders that can complicate or be confused with IBD in the elderly is essential. Although comprehensive reviews of the many different disorders discussed here are available elsewhere, the intent of this article is to provide knowledge specific to IBDs in the elderly population.

EPIDEMIOLOGY
Incidence

Ten percent of patients diagnosed with IBD are older than 60 years of age with an equal distribution between CD and UC.[2,3] Of these about half are diagnosed between 60 and 69 years of age. The true incidence in the elderly is difficult to determine because of differences in populations studied, case definitions of IBD, and potential confusion with other diagnoses such as ischemic colitis or nonsteroidal anti-inflammatory drug (NSAID)-induced colitis. Incidence in Olmsted County, Minnesota increased from 1950 to the 1970s but has stabilized thereafter with rates of 7.9 and 8.8 per 100,000 for CD and UC, respectively.[2–4] The highest incidence was in the 20- to 39-year age group. Rates for UC were consistently higher in men after 1960 compared with women whereas for CD there was no gender difference. Incidence remained stable after age 39, suggesting that there was no bimodal distribution for either disorder. Higher IBD incidence rates were reported in Manitoba, Canada probably because of differences in case ascertainment but rates again were highest in the

Department of Medicine, Division of Gastroenterology, 4500 San Pablo Rd., Mayo Clinic, Jacksonville, FL 32224, USA
* Corresponding author.
E-mail address: picco.michael@mayo.edu (M.F. Picco).

Gastroenterol Clin N Am 38 (2009) 447–462
doi:10.1016/j.gtc.2009.06.006
0889-8553/09/$ – see front matter © 2009 Elsevier Inc. All rights reserved.

20- to 29-year age group for CD and the 20- to 39-year age group for UC.[5] Rates declined progressively with age thereafter in CD and also in UC, but only for women.

Similar trends in incidence were found from population-based studies from Northern France, Germany, and Sweden, where again a bimodal distribution could not be demonstrated.[6–8] However, in a nationwide French study incidence was increased in the 75- to 79-year age group for CD only but the magnitude was small.[9] This newer data contradict older studies that have reported a significant bimodal distribution for age at onset for both UC and CD.[10–15] These earlier studies had less strict criteria for making the diagnosis of IBD that included radiographic findings and gross appearance at endoscopy or surgery. In 81 patients who developed symptoms after age 50 who were labeled as having colitis, three quarters had ischemic colitis, suggesting that misclassification resulted in an artificial secondary peak in the incidence of IBD.[16] Newer studies are enhanced by better case ascertainment because of more improved methods to diagnose IBD.

Although there are differences among populations studied, there are consistent findings in the incidence of IBD across the age spectrum. Among patients older than 40 years, CD incidence seems to decline dramatically from younger populations but remains similar among all later age groups. UC incidence also declines but at a lower rate in older age groups. Although the notion of a bimodal distribution of incidence in IBD remains controversial, it has not been adequately supported by recent studies.

Mortality

Overall mortality among patients with UC seems not to be higher than the general population.[3,17–19] Furthermore, older age of diagnosis was not associated with higher mortality compared with younger ages[3,20] even among those diagnosed after age 65.[20] The effect of CD on overall mortality is controversial.[21] Whereas some studies suggest a decreased overall survival,[3,22–27] others have shown no effect on mortality.[28,29] Survival differences may become apparent only after longer follow-up. In Olmsted County and Copenhagen, Denmark, increased mortality was seen only after follow-up was extended to 21 and 54 years, respectively.[3,25] The effect of age at diagnosis on mortality is also controversial, with some suggesting an increased mortality risk with increasing age,[26] particularly after age 40 years[27] especially early after diagnosis,[29] whereas others have not confirmed this association.

Overall, there does seem to be an increased mortality among patients with CD especially among those diagnosed at an older age or with very long-standing disease. The magnitude of the risk is relatively small and differences in studies may be due to different populations, calendar times, and lengths of follow-up. Higher mortality in CD compared with UC may be due in part to smoking habits,[30] with CD patients more likely to be active smokers and have a higher overall mortality. As the population ages, further information should become available to definitively answer the question as to the impact of aging on the onset and severity of IBD.

CLINICAL MANIFESTATIONS AND PROGNOSIS
Crohn Disease

CD is a heterogeneous disease that is classified based on age at diagnosis, disease location, and behavior. The Montreal classification[31] (modified from the Vienna classification[32]) considers patient's age at diagnosis as before 16, between 17 and 40, and after age 40 years. Disease presentation among individuals diagnosed after the age of 40 (mean 52.2 years) was similar to those diagnosed before age 40 (mean 24 years).[33]

Early reports suggested a higher proportion of isolated colonic disease with a propensity for the rectum and sigmoid in those older than 55 to 60 years of age.[34–36] Prognosis was variable, which may have been because of small numbers of patients, differences in presentation and treatment, and misclassification of other disorders such as ischemic colitis or diverticular colitis as CD (**Table 1**).

Subsequent studies from referral centers have found that the proportion of patients with colonic involvement increases with increasing age at diagnosis.[37,38] Of those diagnosed after age 40, 48% had isolated colonic involvement compared with 28% and 20% for those diagnosed between age 20 and 40 and before age 20, respectively.[38] In a population-based study from Brittany from 2004, 66% of patients diagnosed at 60 years of age or older had isolated colonic involvement.[39] Furthermore, the proportion of patients with inflammatory (nonstricturing, nonpenetrating) behavior also increased among those diagnosed after age 40. Although overall probabilities for surgery were similar between patients older and younger than 60 years, azathioprine use and the likelihood for hospitalization from a second flare were lower in those diagnosed after age 60. These 3 studies suggest that isolated colon disease is more common in community than referral populations and is less severe among elderly patients.

Ulcerative Colitis

Although rectal bleeding and diarrhea remain the most common presentation of UC at any age, older patients (more than 50 years old) with ulcerative colitis may rarely present with atypical symptoms such as constipation.[40] Younger patients tended to have more severe symptoms of diarrhea, fever, and weight loss but differences between older and younger patients were minimal. Older patients tended to have proctocolitis and younger patients extensive colitis.[40,41] The first attack of colitis tended to be more severe in those older than age 50, with longer duration of symptoms and greater likelihood of needing oral corticosteroids.[41,42] Overall, advanced patient age was not associated with overall poorer quality of life.[42] Better quality of life was associated with lack of clinical symptoms and longer duration of disease, suggesting that patients may adjust to their illness (**Table 1**).

INFLAMMATORY BOWEL DISEASE: TREATMENT
Medical Therapy

Unfortunately, there are few data that directly compare treatment in older and younger patients but it is seems that outcomes are similar.[43] The treatment of CD and UC is

Table 1 Differences in presentation of inflammatory bowel disease in older populations		
	Crohn Disease (Age at Diagnosis ≥40 Years)	**Ulcerative Colitis (Age at Diagnosis ≥50 Years**
Symptoms	No difference compared with patients with similar distribution and behavior	May be less severe with some having atypical symptoms such as constipation
Disease distribution	Isolated colonic disease (typically nonstricturing, nonpenetrating) more common	Distal left-sided or proctosigmoiditis more common
Severity	No difference compared with patients with similar distribution and behavior	First attack often more severe

discussed in detail elsewhere based on clinical disease severity, location and for Crohn disease, and disease behavior.[44–46] This review focuses on IBD treatment issues in the elderly.

Mesalamine is the mainstay of therapy for mild to moderate UC. All forms are equally effective but osalazine may cause diarrhea in some patients. Mesalamine suppositories, and enemas alone or in combination with oral mesalamine are effective among UC patients with proctitis (suppositories), proctosigmoiditis, or left-sided colitis. Older patients may have difficulty retaining suppositories or enemas because of difficulties with continence due to a compromised anal sphincter. Fecal incontinence is common in the general geriatric population with rates as high as 10% to 25% in hospitalized and 4% in outpatient geriatric patients.[47] Continence may be further compromised by rectal inflammation with difficulties becoming apparent only after starting therapy. If enema retention is a problem, the volume of the enema can be decreased and patients still benefit. Other options for topical therapy include hydrocortisone enemas for proctosigmoiditis or left-sided colitis, and hydrocortisone foam for proctitis. Foam preparations are better retained, resulting in less incontinence.

Mesalamine therapy is generally not effective in CD although it may have a role in mild to moderately active Crohn colitis. Antibiotics, though not useful in UC, are beneficial in some cases of CD. Metronidazole is effective among some patients with colonic CD, as postoperative treatment to prevent recurrence following ileocolic resection and in the management of fistula. Unfortunately, side effects often lead to discontinuation of this medication. The most concerning is sensory peripheral neuropathy, which is most commonly associated with chronic use but can also occur when high doses are given for short periods.[48] This requires a careful discussion with the patient and vigilant monitoring. Before starting therapy, a careful history should be taken to exclude preexisting neuropathy because, though generally infrequent, it is more common in the elderly at rates of about 4% after age 55. Preexisting neuropathy is typically seen in association with diabetes but can have multiple causes.[49] In patients with preexisting neuropathy, metronidazole should be avoided. Ciprofloxacin is tolerated better but definitive data on its use are lacking. An extremely rare complication of ciprofloxacin is Achilles tendon rupture, with risk increasing with age and corticosteroid use.[50]

For UC patients who fail mesalamine or have moderate to severe disease, and for those with active CD, parenteral or oral corticosteroids are effective. However, among hospitalized CD patients corticosteroid therapy was associated with a longer length of stay in those older than 50 years, and this persisted after adjustment for disease severity.[51] These medications lead to more adverse effects in elderly populations including osteoporosis, bone fractures, changes in mental status, diabetes, and hypertension.[51,52] Osteoporosis risk is increased in the elderly especially among those with chronic inflammatory disorders like UC and CD and those taking corticosteroids.[53] For IBD overall, prevalence has been estimated at 15%. The Crohn's and Colitis Foundation of America has recommended testing for osteoporosis by dual-energy x-ray absorptiometry at diagnosis of IBD and repeated 12 to 18 months later.[54] Further assessments should be made based on the patient's clinical course and continued need for corticosteroids.

Enteric release budesonide has replaced mesalamine as a first-line medication for the induction remission of mild to moderate CD involving the terminal ileum or ascending colon. Budesonide works topically and has a high first-pass metabolism in the liver, minimizing but not eliminating steroid-related side effects. There is no information available on differences in efficacy and toxicity among older and younger patients.

Among patients receiving corticosteroids, immunomodulator therapy is typically started to facilitate corticosteroid weaning and maintain disease remission. For UC and CD, azathioprine or 6-mercaptopurine is effective for this purpose. These agents require 3 to 4 months of therapy to be effective and there is no evidence of a difference in efficacy, metabolism, or toxicity in older compared with younger patients. However, hematological monitoring is essential in all patients with the potential for significant drug interactions, the most important of which in the elderly is with allopurinol. Allopurinol is more commonly used in the elderly for gout and may result in significant bone marrow toxicity when combined with azathioprine or 6-mercaptopurine. The toxicity is due to inhibition of xanthine oxidase by allopurinol, which is important in the breakdown of these immunomodulators. Despite recommended dosage reductions of azathioprine or 6-mercaptopurine, hematological toxicity has still been reported, underscoring the need for vigilant monitoring.[55] Parenteral methotrexate is also useful as a primary treatment or to facilitate corticosteroid weaning in CD, and there is no evidence for differing efficacy among older and younger age groups. Liver toxicity with this agent may be more important in the elderly due to the greater potential for preexisting liver disease compared with younger patients.

Over the last 10 years biologic therapies that inhibit tumor necrosis factor α (infliximab, adalumimab, and certiluzimab) have revolutionized the management of IBD. These drugs are very effective in the induction and maintenance of remission and are attractive alternatives to oral or parenteral corticosteroids in nonstricturing, nonpenetrating CD. Infliximab and adalumimab are also proven effective in penetrating (fistulizing) CD and infliximab in UC. There is no evidence currently that the efficacy of these agents is altered by subject's age or age at diagnosis. Infliximab is also used in rheumatoid arthritis and in one report there was a trend toward more severe infections requiring discontinuation among patients older than 70 years.[56] However, this was not demonstrated in a randomized trial.[57]

Due to the complexities of management of IBD, patients are often taking combinations of medications including corticosteroids, immunomodulators, biologic agents, or narcotics. The determination of toxicities of individual agents is difficult because of small numbers of subjects. However, Lichtenstein and colleagues[58] developed a registry of 6290 CD patients with 3179 having been administered infliximab to determine the risk of toxicity. In a multivariate analysis, age and duration of disease were associated with a slight increase in mortality rates. However, the strongest influence on mortality was prednisone use, which increased the odds of death two-fold. Furthermore, prednisone and narcotic use each resulted in a two-fold increase in severe infections. Infliximab did not increase mortality or the risk of severe opportunistic infections.

Surgical Therapy

Surgery for CD is not curative, and is indicated for failure of medical therapy or the development of complications.[59] Complications include perforation with abscess or fistula formation and obstruction. Malignancy may occur, especially in long-standing colitis, and is treated by total colectomy with ileostomy formation. The risk of surgery for nonneoplastic bowel disease decreases with age.[60] Age at diagnosis older than 40 years and colonic disease (a location common in the elderly) were independently associated with lower rates of surgery.[61] Older patients with isolated ileocecal disease had similar rates of resection to younger patients.[62]

Surgery for UC is curative, and is typically performed for colonic dysplasia or treatment of refractory disease.[63] Complete colectomy with ileal pouch-anal anastomosis (IPAA) is the preferred surgery in most patients. IPAA is usually performed as a two-stage procedure with the first stage being total colectomy, pouch construction, and diverting ileostomy, and the second stage being takedown of the diverting ileostomy about 3 months later. A permanent end-ileostomy (without an ileoanal pouch) is more appropriate in some patients. The decision on which operation to perform depends on the indication for the procedure and patient-specific factors.

Some studies have shown a marginally higher morbidity as measured by symptom index, and higher rates of fecal incontinence and stool frequency in patients older than 45 or 50 years.[64–66] However, the overwhelming majority of older patients were satisfied with their result. Pouch failure rates between younger and older patients were similar as were rates of pouchitis. These studies are representative of a body of literature that led The American Society of Colon and Rectal Surgeons to recommend that "chronologic age should not itself be an exclusion criterion" for IPAA.[63] Optimal patient selection is important, restricting this operation to motivated patients, without significant cognitive problems or compromised anal sphincter function.

INFLAMMATORY BOWEL DISEASE: COLORECTAL CANCER

The most important risk factors for colon cancer among patients with UC (and CD colitis) are disease duration and extent, with the highest risk in those with long-standing pancolitis.[67–69] The following discussion also applies to Crohn colitis. Older age at diagnosis is not a risk factor for UC- related colon cancer. Current medical therapy is effective at staving off colectomy but the risk of colorectal cancer continues to increase with time. The key to altering outcome is in early detection of dysplasia, the precancerous change in UC, by colonoscopy with biopsies every 1 to 2 years. This process begins after 8 years of pancolitis and 10 to 15 years of left-sided colitis whereby the risks of cancer development become significant. Proctitis is not associated with an increased risk. Unlike sporadic colon cancers that result from the standard adenoma carcinoma sequence, UC-related cancers develop in a background of colonic inflammation and regeneration.[67–70] Unlike adenomas (the precancerous lesion in non-UC cancers) that can be seen by colonoscopy, the precancerous lesion in UC typically occurs as a flat patch not readily apparent at colonoscopy.

Unfortunately, current surveillance methods predominately rely on multiple colonic biopsies (at least 32) in the hope of picking up dysplasia, but are imperfect. Pathologists divide dysplasia into low-grade (LGD) and high-grade dysplasia (HGD). The degree of dysplasia predicts the likelihood of colorectal cancer development in the future and the presence of coexisting malignancy that was not apparent during the colonoscopy. Colectomy is recommended for the finding of any dysplasia.

Current methods of surveillance using white light endoscopy alone are imperfect, cumbersome, and expensive.[71,72] Chromoscopy involves the spray application of dye solutions, typically indigo carmine or methylene blue, to the colonic mucosa, improving dysplasia detection.[73–75] Chromoscopy is recommended in United States surveillance guidelines for the dysplasia detection in UC,[76] but this practice has not gained broad acceptance.

The risk of developing sporadic colon polyps increases with age. In fact, among the general population aged 48 to 62 years who undergo screening colonoscopy, 9% to 18% will have adenomas detected.[77] With advances in therapy for UC, patients are keeping their colons longer, increasing their risk of dysplasia but also increasing the likelihood that they will develop sporadic (not related to UC) polyps. Such sporadic polyps may be confused with the more ominous dysplasia-associated lesion or mass (DALM) that would indicate HGD and require colectomy.

The ability to differentiate between a sporadic polyp and a DALM lesion was addressed in two studies suggesting that simple polypectomy was sufficient among lesions characterized as sporadic polyps, with no resulting malignancy after 4 years.[78,79] Characteristics that suggested a sporadic polyp were a lesion outside the area of histologically evident colitis, a pedunculated lesion or discrete nodule (ie, not carpet-like), short duration of disease, no dysplasia around the polyp, or the absence of primary sclerosing cholangitis. With these criteria, nearly 50% had recurrent polyps with further surveillance in both studies, only one patient developed a DALM at follow-up, and there were no malignancies. Although the number of patients followed was small, the findings did suggest that for a lesion that meets the criteria for a sporadic polyp, a conservative approach of simple polypectomy followed by careful continued surveillance may spare some patients colectomy. However, more data are needed before this approach can be endorsed in all patients. The finding of a colon "polyp" in a patient with long-standing UC remains a dilemma for clinicians and the decision for colectomy should be based on clinical findings, the patient's suitability for colectomy, and their preference after discussion of risk and clinical uncertainty.

DIFFERENTIAL DIAGNOSIS AND COMPLICATING CONDITIONS

The diagnosis of IBD can be particularly difficult in elderly patients. IBD can be complicated by infection and medications, or be confused with other conditions including microscopic colitis, NSAID-induced colitis, diverticular colitis, or ischemic colitis (**Table 2**). Malignancy, particularly lymphoma of the small bowel, is a particular concern in older age groups because it can mimic the features of IBD or complicate existing IBD. Although techniques have improved, diagnosis of malignancy may still

Table 2
Common causes of chronic diarrhea and bowel inflammation in the elderly

	Common Presentations in the Elderly	Specific Issues in Elderly Populations
Clostridium difficile infection	Watery or bloody diarrhea that may cause fever	Highest carriage, infection, morbidity and mortality in those older than 65 years
Microscopic colitis	Watery diarrhea without bleeding or fever. Wide range of severity most common after age 50	Cause of 20% of chronic diarrhea in those older than 70 years. May be associated with celiac disease
Diverticular colitis	Rectal bleeding, abdominal pain, bowel habit changes most common after age 60	Segmental colitis in an area of diverticula that can be confused with Crohn disease
Nonsteroidal anti-inflammatory drug-induced colitis	Wide variety of signs and symptoms including rectal bleeding, abdominal pain, obstruction, or bowel perforation	Can mimic inflammatory bowel disease or bowel ischemia. Leads to worsening existing Crohn disease or ulcerative colitis
Ischemic colitis	Abrupt onset of pain and bloody diarrhea	Segmental colitis in "watershed areas" of colon. Inciting factor may not be found in elderly patients

be difficult and clinical suspicion must remain high. Other conditions such as amyloidosis, vasculitis, and radiation enteritis should also be considered in some patients.

Infection

Gastrointestinal infections are an important cause of diarrhea in the elderly that result in significant morbidity and mortality. In a comparison of healthy individuals aged 21 to 34 years with those aged 67 to 88 years, the older patients had alterations in the concentrations of "probiotic bacteria" (bifidobacteria and lactobacilli) that could increase the risk of enteric infections.[80] Common source outbreaks are more likely to occur in nursing homes or assisted living facilities. Among all patients presenting with diarrhea including those with known IBD, routine studies should be performed to exclude common infectious pathogens such as *Salmonella*, *Shigella*, *Campylobacter*, and *Clostridium difficile*. Other less common pathogens should be excluded based on clinical presentation. *Yersinia enterocolitica*, for example, may result in ileitis and mimic IBD. Clinical laboratories vary in what is tested for in routine stool samples so clinicians may need to make specific requests for pathogens when suspected. This is particularly true of *Escherichia coli* O157:H7, which is a common cause of bloody diarrhea that can result in significant morbidity and mortality.

Among enteric pathogens, geriatric patients are more susceptible to *C difficile*. The clinical presentation of *C difficile*-associated disease (CDAD) can vary from watery diarrhea to fulminant colitis. From 2000 to 2005 in the United States there was a 23% annual increase in CDAD hospitalizations.[81] The case fatality rate doubled from 1.2% in 2000 to 2.3% in 2004 due to increased virulence of the organism. Rates were highest and increased most dramatically in those older than 65 years. Infection with a newer hypervirulent strain prolonged hospitalization by 11 days and had a 30-day mortality of 23% compared with 7% in a control group adjusted for age and comorbidity.[82] Rates of asymptomatic carriage increase with age, and are up to 13% in the hospital setting.[83]

IBD (CD or UC) increases the risk of CDAD.[84] Incidence of CDAD among hospitalized IBD patients doubled for CD and tripled for UC from 1998 to 2004.[85] The majority of infections were acquired before hospitalization. CDAD pursues a more aggressive course among IBD patients resulting in a higher rate of complications and 4 times the mortality compared with those admitted for IBD alone.[84,86] These findings underscore the need for a high level of suspicion among all patients with IBD presenting with diarrhea, even in the absence of antibiotic exposure or hospitalization.

Microscopic Colitis

Microscopic colitis (MC) is a chronic inflammatory disease of the colon that is an important cause of chronic watery diarrhea in the elderly. MC is separated into lymphocytic (LC) and collagenous colitis (CC), based on histology with a grossly normal colonoscopy. CC is much more common in women. MC is the cause in 10% of all patients and up to 20% of those older than 70 years of age presenting with chronic diarrhea.[87] Overall population incidence rates from both Europe and the United States vary from 1.8 to 7.1 per 100,000 for LC and 4.4 to 12.6 per 100,000 for CC.[87–92] The higher rates are from more recent studies, probably because of a lower threshold for colonoscopy with biopsy due to a greater physician awareness of this condition. This improvement also may in part be explained by increasing overall rates of colonoscopy and sigmoidoscopy with time.[92]

The incidence of MC increases with age most dramatically after age 50 years,[89] and diagnosis is usually made in the sixth or seventh decade of life. Patients older than 65 years are two times as likely to be diagnosed with MC compared with those younger than 65, with incidence rates of more than 30 per 100,000.[88] Whether this represents a true increase in incidence in older populations or a lower threshold for colonoscopy is not clear. Although 10% of patients with MC will have celiac disease,[87,88,92] in the absence of findings of malabsorption routine testing for celiac disease is not recommended.[93] MC has also been associated with hypothyroidism. Despite the chronic inflammation in MC there seems to be no increased risk of colon cancer based on a series of patients with CC followed for 7 years.[94]

The clinical course of MC is variable with treatment aimed at controlling symptoms. In mild cases avoidance of offending foods alone or with antidiarrheal medications will control symptoms. As severity increases, medication therapies such as mesalamine, enteric released budesonide, or systemic corticosteroids may be needed.[93] Rarely immunomodulators or a colectomy may be necessary. Older patients may have a more benign course with a greater likelihood of spontaneous remission and more easily controlled disease, as suggested by a lower use of mesalamine and corticosteroids.[95]

Among patients requiring mesalamine or corticosteroids, 23% and 54%, respectively were taking NSAIDs compared with only 6% managed with no treatment or antidiarrheal therapy only. However, withdrawal of NSAIDs did not lead to improvement. This result is in contrast to reports of improvement with discontinuation of NSAIDs[96] and recurrence of symptoms with rechallenge. In one case report, diarrhea ceased and histologic changes reversed when aspirin was discontinued.[97] Others have found no association of NSAIDs with development of MC.[98] All of these studies suffer from small sample size, limiting their conclusions. Overall the existing evidence does suggest a role for NSAIDs in the development and worsening course in MC. Given the higher proportion of elderly with MC and the higher rates of NSAID use compared with younger populations, these medications in the setting of MC should be avoided.

Diverticular Colitis

Diverticulosis affects more than half of individuals older than 60 years[99] and is described elsewhere in this issue. Diverticular colitis is an important cause of rectal bleeding, abdominal pain, and change in bowel habit, but is relatively uncommon, with only 3% developing inflammation in the mucosa surrounding diverticuli.[100] Segmental colitis presents in individuals older than 60 years and can mimic the endoscopic and histologic appearance of CD.[101–103] The inflammation is confined to the segment containing the diverticula with the rectum and uninvolved bowel having normal endoscopic appearance and histology. A nonspecific chronic colitis that may contain granulomas is seen on histology, further adding to the confusion with CD. However, diverticular colitis represents a distinct clinical entity separate from CD as evident from natural history studies, and is independent of classic diverticulitis.

Unfortunately, there are no randomized treatment studies for diverticular colitis and recommendations are based on reports from relatively few patients.[102,104] Among 19 patients, 14 responded to conservative therapy with high fiber diet or antibiotics, with failures responding to sulfasalazine (three patients) or sulfasalazine and steroid enemas (two patients).[105] Most patients treated with mesalamine have excellent results. Response rates of 80% within 6 months were reported among 21 patients taking oral mesalamine.[104] Five patients who initially responded but were not compliant with this therapy relapsed, with three responding to further mesalamine and two requiring prednisone. Response rates were 100% among 14 patients treated with 2.4 g/d of oral mesalamine and 2 g/d of mesalamine enema at 6 weeks.[106] In these 14 patients therapy was stopped and only one patient had clinical and endoscopic relapse at 1 year. Whereas a conservative approach may be effective in some patients, oral and topical mesalamine therapy seems to provide the best long-term response rate among patients with diverticular colitis. For patients who do not respond to conservative therapy, antibiotics, or mesalamine, steroid enemas may provide benefit, with only the minority of patients requiring surgery.

Nonsteroidal Anti-Inflammatory Medications

Although many different medications can cause gastrointestinal inflammation, the most common and arguably the most important are NSAIDs. NSAIDs can cause a myriad of complications in the small and the large intestine from ulceration or bleeding to perforation or stricture.[107,108] Mucosal findings may range from acute inflammation to chronic nonspecific inflammation with fibrosis. Perforation can also occur, especially among patients with diverticulosis.

The strongest association of NSAIDs among the IBDs is with UC and CD. UC patients who relapsed were twice as likely to be using chronic NSAIDs.[109] Subsequent studies[110,111] have supported these findings. Rate of relapse was increased to 20% for UC and CD when patients were treated with a nonselective cyclooxygenase inhibitor (COX) or conventional NSAID for 4 weeks.[112] Most patients relapsed within 9 days of starting these medications. No patients treated with acetaminophen relapsed. Patients assigned to acetaminophen, nimesulide (a selective COX-2 inhibitor), or aspirin (a selective COX-1 inhibitor) had lower rates of relapse than those taking nonselective agents.

In a randomized study comparing celecoxib (selective COX-2 inhibitor) to placebo among patients with UC in remission, rates of relapse over 14 days were similar, at 3% and 4%, respectively.[113] All patients were taking maintenance therapy with mesalamine or azathioprine/6-mercaptopurine. It was not clear if the dose of celecoxib in this study adequately treated the arthritis or arthropathy in this population, but it does represent a standard dose. Furthermore, rofecoxib has been associated with cardiovascular risk[114] and has been withdrawn whereas celecoxib results regarding this toxicity have been conflicting,[115,116] leading to caution in its use among clinicians.

Arthralgias and arthritis remain common complaints in the elderly and also among those with IBD. Peripheral arthritis from IBD usually responds to treatment of the underlying active inflammatory bowel disease. Axillary arthritis such as ankylosing spondylitis and sacroileitis typically does not. Whereas occasional use of an NSAID is probably safe, many patients require long-term pain control that may not respond to acetaminophen. In these patients, unfortunately, clinicians have few effective options, leading to the decision to use NSAIDs in these patients when the benefit to quality of life outweighs the risks. Although selective COX-2 inhibitors may provide a better option, the evidence is not clear and cardiovascular toxicity needs to be considered in prescribing these agents.

Ischemic Colitis

Ischemic colitis is a common condition in the elderly with an average age at presentation of 68 years[117] and is discussed elsewhere in this issue. Ischemic colitis results from an interruption of blood supply to the colon causing a segmental colitis that can be confused with CD.[118] Areas affected tend to be "watershed areas" that are more susceptible to sparing of the rectum due to its rich blood supply. There are multiple causes of this condition including cardiac failure, thromboembolic disease, hypercoagulable states, and medications.

Most patients present with the abrupt onset of pain and bloody diarrhea with typical findings of segmental colitis on computed tomography that can be confirmed by colonoscopy with biopsy. Care is largely supportive with the minority of patients requiring surgery. Biopsy, clinical presentation, and course are all useful in distinguishing this entity from other IBDs. Full colonoscopy should be strongly considered to exclude malignancy, a rare but important cause of this presentation especially in the elderly.

SUMMARY

IBD will grow in prevalence as the population ages. Prognosis of late-onset UC is generally similar to that of early-onset UC, whereas in CD it is probably better because of a tendency for colonic involvement. Disease complications are related more to the duration of the IBD than the subject's current age. The diagnosis in elderly patients can be challenging due to the large number of conditions that mimic IBD on radiologic, endoscopic, and histologic testing. Distinguishing these conditions from IBD will significantly alter prognosis and treatment. Complications related to IBD and its treatment are common and must be recognized early to limit their impact in a vulnerable elderly population.

REFERENCES

1. Robertson DJ, Grimm IS. Inflammatory bowel disease in the elderly. Gastroenterol Clin North Am 2001;30:409–26.
2. Loftus EV, Silverstein MD, Sandborn WJ, et al. Crohn's disease in Olmsted county Minnesota 1940–1993: incidence, prevalence and survival. Gastroenterol 1998;114:1161–8.
3. Loftus EV, Silverstein MD, Sandborn WJ, et al. Ulcerative colitis in Olmsted county Minnesota 1940–1993: incidence, prevalence and survival. Gut 2000; 200(46):336–43.
4. Loftus CG, Loftus EV, Harmsen S, et al. Update on the incidence and prevalence of Crohn's disease and ulcerative colitis in Olmsted county, Minnesota, 1940–2000. Inflamm Bowel Dis 2007;13:254–61.
5. Bernstein CN, Blanchard JF, Rawsthorne P, et al. Epidemiology of Crohn's disease and ulcerative colitis in a central Canadian province: a population based study. Am J Epidemiol 1999;149:916–24.
6. Molinie F, Gower-Rousseau C, Yzet T, et al. Opposite evolution in incidence of Crohn's disease and ulcerative colitis in Northern France. Gut 2004;53:843–8.
7. Ott C, Obermeier F, Thieler S, et al. The incidence of inflammatory bowel disease in Southern Germany: a prospective population based study. Eur J Gastroenterol Hepatol 2008;20:917–23.
8. Lapidus A, Bernell O, Hellers G, et al. Incidence of Crohn's disease in Stockholm County 1955-1989. Gut 1997;41:480–6.
9. Nerich V, Monnet E, Etienne A, et al. Geographical variations of inflammatory bowel disease in France: a study based on national health insurance data. Inflamm Bowel Dis 2006;218–26.
10. Evans JG, Acheson ED. An epidemiological study of ulcerative colitis and regional enteritis in the Oxford area. Gut 1965;6:311–24.
11. Burch PR, de Dombal FT, Watkinson G. Aetiology of ulcerative colitis. II. A new hypothesis. Gut 1969;10:277–84.
12. Lee F, Costello FT. Crohn's disease in Blackpool—incidence and prevalence 1968-80. Gut 1985;26:274–8.
13. Terrell KB, Garland FC. Incidence rates of ulcerative colitis and Crohn's disease in fifteen areas of the United States. Gastroenterology 1981;81:1115–24.

14. Garland CF, Lilienfeld AM, Mendeloff AI, et al. Incidence rates of ulcerative colitis and Crohn's disease in fifteen areas of the United States. Gastroenterology 1981;81:1115–24.

15. Rose JDR, Roberts GM, Williams RG. Cardiff Crohn's disease jubilee: the incidence over 50 years. Gut 1988;29:346–51.

16. Brandt L. Colitis in the elderly. A reappraisal. Am J Gastroenterol 1981;76: 239–45.

17. Hendriksen C, Kreiner S, Binder V. Long term prognosis in ulcerative colitis-based on results from regional patient group from the county of Copenhagen. Gut 1985;26:158–63.

18. Sonnenberg A. Mortality of Crohn's disease and ulcerative colitis in England-Wales and the U.S. from 1950 to 1983. Dis Colon Rectum 1986;29:624–9.

19. Stonnington CM, Phillips SF, Zinsmeister AR. Prognosis in chronic ulcerative colitis in a community. Gut 1987;28:1261–6.

20. Jones HW, Hoare AM. Does ulcerative colitis behave differently in the elderly? Age Ageing 1988;17:410–4.

21. Loftus E. A matter of life or death: Mortality in Crohn's disease. Inflamm Bowel Dis 2002;8:428–9.

22. Palli D, Trallori G, Saieva C, et al. General and cancer specific mortality of a population based cohort of patients with inflammatory bowel disease: the Florence study. Gut 1998;42:175–9.

23. Ekbom A, Helmick CG, Zack M, et al. Survival and causes of death in patients with inflammatory bowel disease: a population based study. Gastroenterology 1992;103:954–60.

24. Persson PG, Bernell O, Leijonmarck CE, et al. Survival and cause-specific mortality in inflammatory bowel disease: a population based cohort study. Gastroenterology 1996;110:1339–45.

25. Jess T, Winther KV, Munkholm P. Mortality and causes of death in Crohn's disease. Follow-up of a population-based cohort in Copenhagen county, Denmark. Gastroenterology 2002;122:1808–14.

26. Jess T, Loftus EV, Harmsen WS, et al. Survival and cause specific mortality in patients with inflammatory bowel disease: a long term outcome study in Olmsted County, Minnesota, Gut 2006;55:1248–54.

27. Wolters FL, Russel MG, Sijbrandij J, et al. Crohn's disease: increased mortality 10 years after diagnosis in a Europe-wide population based cohort. Gut 2006; 55:510–8.

28. Probert CSJ, Jayanthi V, Wicks ACB, et al. Mortality from Crohn's disease in Leicestershire, 1972–1989: an epidemiological community based study. Gut 1992;33:1226–8.

29. Farrokhyar F, Swarbrick ET, Grace RH, et al. Low mortality in ulcerative colitis and Crohn's disease in three regional centers in England. Am J Gastroenterol 2001;96:501–7.

30. Masala G, Bagnoli S, Ceroti M, et al. Divergent patterns of total cancer mortality in ulcerative colitis and Crohn's disease patients: the Florence IBD study 1978-2001. Gut 2004;53:1309–13.

31. Satsangi J, Silverberg Ms, Vermeire S, et al. The Montreal classification of inflammatory bowel disease: controversies, consensus and implications. Gut 2006;55: 749–53.

32. Gasche C, Scholmerich J, Brynskov J. A simple classification of Crohn's disease: report of the working party for the World Congress of Gastroenterology, Vienna 1998. Inflamm Bowel Dis 2000;6:8–15.

33. Wagtmans MJ, Verspaget HW, Lamers C, et al. Crohn's disease in the elderly: a comparison with young adults. J Clin Gastroenterol 1998;27:129–33.
34. Fabricius PJ, Gynde SN, Shouler P, et al. Crohn's disease in the elderly. Gut 1985;26:461–5.
35. Stalnikowicz R, Eliakim R, Diab R, et al. Crohn's disease in the elderly. J Clin Gastroenterol 1989;11:411–5.
36. Walmsley RS, Gillen CD, Allan RN. Prognosis and management of Crohn's disease in the over-55 age group. Postgrad Med J 1997;73:225–9.
37. Polito J, Childs B, Mellits D, et al. Crohn's disease: influence of age at diagnosis on site and clinical type of disease. Gastroenterology 1996;11:580–6.
38. Freeman HJ. Age-dependent phenotypic clinical expression of Crohn's disease. J Clin Gastroenterol 2005;39:774–7.
39. Heresbach D, Alexandre J-L, Bretagne JF, et al. Crohn's disease in the over 60 age group: a population based study. Eur J Gastroenterol Hepatol 2004;16:657–64.
40. Riegler G, Tartaglione MT, Carratu R, et al. Age-related clinical severity at diagnosis in 1705 patients with ulcerative colitis: a study by GISC (Italian Colon-Rectum Study Group). Dig Dis Sci 2000;45:462–5.
41. Zimmerman J, Gavish D, Rachmilewitz D. Early and late onset ulcerative colitis: distinct clinical features. J Clin Gastroenterol 1985;7:492–8.
42. Han SW, McColl E, Barton JR. Predictors of quality of life in ulcerative colitis. The importance of symptoms and illness representations. Inflamm Bowel Dis 2005; 11:24–34.
43. Pardi DS, Loftus EV, Camilleri M. Treatment of inflammatory bowel disease in the elderly. An update. Drugs Ageing 2002;19:355–63.
44. Lichtenstein GR, Hanauer SB, Sandborn WJ. Management of Crohn's disease in adults. Am J Gastroenterol 2009;104:465–83.
45. Brain O, Travis SPL. Therapy for ulcerative colitis: state of the art. Curr Opin Gastroenterol 2008;469–74.
46. Kornbluth A, Sachar DB. Ulcerative colitis practice guidelines in adults. Am J Gastroenterol 1997;92:204–11.
47. Rao SSC. Diagnosis and management of fecal incontinence. Am J Gastroenterol 2004;99:1585–604.
48. Duffy LF, Daum F, Fisher SE, et al. Peripheral neuropathy in Crohn's disease patients treated with metronidazole. Gastroenterology 1985;88:681–4.
49. Italian General Practitioner Study Group. Chronic symmetric symptomatic poly-neuropathy in the elderly: a field screening investigation of two Italian regions. I. Prevalence and general characteristics of the sample. Neurology 1995;45: 1832–6.
50. Casparian JM, Luchi M, Moffat RE. Quinolones and tendon ruptures. Southampt Med J 2000;93:488–91.
51. Thomas TP. The complications of systemic corticosteroid therapy in the elderly. A retrospective study. Gerontology 1984;30:60–5.
52. Akerkar GA, Peppercorn MA, Hamel MB. Corticosteroid-associated complications in elderly Crohn's disease patients. Am J Gastroenterol 1997;92:461–4.
53. Tilg H, Moschen AR, Kaser A, et al. Gut inflammation and osteoporosis: basic and clinical concepts. Gut 2008;57:684–94.
54. Lichtenstein GR, Sands BE, Pazianas M. Prevention and treatment of osteoporosis in inflammatory bowel disease. Inflamm Bowel Dis 2006;12:797–813.
55. Cummins D, Sekar M, Halil O. Myelosuprression associated with azathioprine-allopurinol interaction after heart and lung transplantation. Transplantation 1996;61:1661–2.

56. Chevillotte-Mallard H, Orneti P, Mistrich R, et al. Survival and safety of treatment with infliximab in the elderly population. Rheumatology 2005;44:695–6.

57. Mani R, St Clair EW, Breedveld F, et al. Infliximab (chimeric anti-tumour necrosis factor alpha monoclonal antibody) versus placebo in rheumatoid arthritis patients receiving concomitant methotrexate: a randomized phase III trial. ATTRACT Study Group. Lancet 1999;354:1932–9.

58. Lichtenstein GR, Feagan BG, Cohen RD, et al. Serious infections and mortality in association with therapies for Crohn's disease: TREAT registry. Clin Gastroenterol Hepatol 2006;4:621–30.

59. Strong SA, Koltun WA, Hyman NH. Practice parameters for the surgical management of Crohn's disease. Dis Colon Rectum 2007;50:1735–46.

60. Tremaine WJ, Tommons LJ, Loftus EV, et al. Age at onset of inflammatory bowel disease and the risk of surgery for non-neoplastic bowel disease. Aliment Pharmacol Ther 2007;25:1435–41.

61. Wolters FL, Russel MG, Sijbrandij J, et al. Phenotype at diagnosis predicts recurrence rates in Crohn's disease. Gut 2006;55:1124–30.

62. Bernell O, Lapidus A, Hellers G. Risk factors for surgery and recurrence in 907 patients with primary ileocecal Crohn's disease. Br J Surg 2000;1697–701.

63. Cohen JL, Strong SA, Hyman NH. Practice parameters for the surgical treatment of ulcerative colitis. Dis Colon Rectum 2005;48:1997–2009.

64. Delaney CP, Fazio VW, Remzi FH, et al. Prospective age-related analysis of surgical results, functional outcome, and quality of life after ileal pouch-anal anastomosis. Ann Surg 2003;238:221–8.

65. Karlbom U, Raab Y, Ejerblad S. Factors influencing outcome of restorative proctocolectomy in ulcerative colitis. Br J Surg 2000;87:1401–8.

66. Farouk R, Pemberton JH, Wolff BG, et al. Functional outcomes after ileal pouch-anal anastomosis for chronic ulcerative colitis. Ann Surg 2000;231:919–26.

67. Itzkowitz SH, Yio X. Inflammation and cancer IV. Colorectal cancer in inflammatory bowel disease: the role of inflammation. Am J Physiol Gastrointest Liver Physiol 2004;287(1):G7–17.

68. Munkholm P. Review article: the incidence and prevalence of colorectal cancer in inflammatory bowel disease. Aliment Pharmacol Ther 2003;18(Suppl. 2):1–5.

69. Itzkowitz SH, Harpaz N. Diagnosis and management of dysplasia in patients with inflammatory bowel diseases. Gastroenterology 2004;126(6):1634–48.

70. Coussens LM, Werb Z. Inflammatory cells and cancer: think different!. J Exp Med 2001;193(6):F23–6.

71. Shanahan F, Quera R. CON: surveillance for ulcerative colitis-associated cancer: time to change the endoscopy and the microscopy. Am J Gastroenterol 2004; 99(9):1633–6.

72. Fujii S, Fujimori T, Chiba T, et al. Efficacy of surveillance and molecular markers for detection of ulcerative colitis-associated colorectal neoplasia. J Gastroenterol 2003;38(12):1117–25.

73. Kiesslich R, Neurath MF. Chromoendoscopy and other novel imaging techniques. Gastroenterol Clin North Am 2006;35:605–19.

74. Kiesslich R, Fritsch J, Holtman M, et al. Methylene blue-aided chromoendoscopy for the detection of intraepithelial neoplasia and colon cancer in ulcerative colitis. Gastroenterology 2003;124:880–8.

75. Hurlstone DP, Sanders DS, Lobo AJ, et al. Indigo carmine-assisted high magnification chromoscopic colonoscopy for the detection and characterization of intraepithelial neoplasia in ulcerative colitis: a prospective evaluation. Endoscopy 2005;37:1186–92.

76. Itzkowitz SH, Present DH. Consensus conference: colon cancer screening and surveillance in inflammatory bowel disease. Inflamm Bowel Dis 2005;11:314–21.
77. Kahi CJ, Rex DK, Imperiale TF. Screening, surveillance and primary prevention for colorectal cancer: a review of recent literature. Gastroenterology 2008;135: 380–99.
78. Rubin DH, Friedman H, Harpaz N, et al. Colonoscopic polypectomy in chronic colitis: conservative management after endoscopic resection of dysplastic polyps. Gastroenterology 1999;117:1295–300.
79. Engelsgjerd M, Farraye F, Odze RD. Polypectomy may be adequate treatment for adenoma-like dysplastic lesions in chronic ulcerative colitis. Gastroenterology 1999;117:1288–94.
80. Hopkins MJ, Macfarlane GT. Changes in predominant bacterial populations in human faeces with age and with *Clostridium difficile* infection. J Med Microbiol 2002;51:448–54.
81. Zilberberg MD, Shorr AF, Kollef M. Increase in adult *Clostridium difficile*-related hospitalizations and case-fatality rate, United States, 2000–2005. Emerg Infect Dis 2006;14:929–31.
82. Pepin J, Valiquette L, Cossette B. Mortality attributable to nosocomial *Clostridium difficile*-associated disease during an epidemic caused by a hyper-virulent strain in Quebec. CMAJ 2005;173:1037–42.
83. McFarland LV, Surawicz CM, Stamm WE. Risk factors for *Clostridium difficile* carriage and C. difficile-associated diarrhea in a cohort of hospitalized patients. J Infect Dis 1990;162:678–84.
84. Issa M, Ananthakrishnan AN, Binion DG. *Clostridium difficile* and inflammatory bowel disease. Inflamm Bowel Dis 2008;14:1432–42.
85. Rodemann JF, Dubberke ER, Reske KA, et al. Incidence of *Clostridium difficile* infection in inflammatory bowel. Clin Gastroenterol Hepatol 2007;5:339–44.
86. Ananthakrishnan AN, McGinley EL, Binion DG. Excess hospitalisation burden associated with *Clostridium difficile* in patients with inflammatory bowel disease. Gut 2008;57:205–10.
87. Olesen M, Eriksson S, Bohr J, et al. Microscopic colitis: A common diarrhoeal disease. An epidemiological in Orebo, Sweden, 1993–1998. Gut 2004;53: 346–50.
88. Williams JJ, Kaplan GG, Makhija S, et al. Microscopic colitis-defining incidence rates and risk factors: a population based study. Clin Gastroenterol Hepatol 2008;6:35–40.
89. Fernandez-Banares F, Salas A, Forne M, et al. Incidence of collagenous and lymphocytic colitis: a 5 year population-based study. Am J Gastroenterol 1999;94:418–23.
90. Bohr J, Tysk C, Eriksson S, et al. Collagenous colitis in Orebo, Sweden, an epidemiological study 1984–1993. Gut 1995;37:394–7.
91. Agnarsdottir M, Gunnlaugsson O, Orvar KB, et al. Collageous and lymphocytic colitis in Ireland. Dig Dis Sci 2002;47:1122–8.
92. Pardi DS, Loftus EV, Smyrk TC, et al. The epidemiology of microscopic colitis: a population based study in Olmsted County, Minnesota. Gut 2007;56:504–8.
93. Pardi DS. Microscopic colitis. An update. Inflamm Bowel Dis 2004;10:860–70.
94. Chan JL, Tersmette AC, Offerhaus GJA, et al. Cancer risk in collagenous colitis. Inflamm Bowel Dis 1999;5:40–3.
95. Abdo A, Raboud J, Freeman HJ, et al. Clinical and histological predictors of response to medical therapy in collagenous colitis. Am J Gastroenterol 2002; 97:1164–8.

96. Riddell RH, Tanaka M, Mazzoleni G. Non-steroidal anti-inflammatory drugs as a possible cause for microscopic colitis: a case control study. Gut 1992;33:683–6.

97. Yagi K, Nakamura A, Sekine A, et al. Nonsteroidal anti-inflammatory drug-associated colitis with histology of collagenous colitis. Endoscopy 2001;33:629–32.

98. Veress B, Lofberg R, Bergman L. Microscopic colitis syndrome. Gut 1995;36:880–6.

99. Manousos ON, Truelove SC, Lumsden K. Prevalence of colonic diverticulosis in the general populationof the Oxford area. Br Med J 1967;3:762–3.

100. Renius JF, Brandt LJ. Vascular ectasias and diverticulosis. Common causes of lower intestinal bleeding. Gastroenterol Clin North Am 1994;23:1–20.

101. Peppercorn MA. Drug-responsive chronic segmental colitis associated with diverticula: a clinical syndrome in the elderly. Am J Gastroenterol 1992;87:609–12.

102. Harpaz N, Sachar DB. Segemental colitis associated with diverticular disease and other IBD look-alikes. J Clin Gastroenterol 2006;40:S132–5.

103. Nielsen OH, Vainer B, Rask-Madden J. Non-IBD and noninfectious colitis. Nat Clin Pract Gastroenterol Hepatol 2008;5:28–39.

104. Freeman HJ. Natural history and long-term clinical behavior of segmental colitis associated with diverticulosis (Scad syndrome). Dig Dis Sci 2008;53:2452–7.

105. Makapugay L, Dean P. Diverticular disease associated colitis. Am J Surg Pathol 1996;20:94–102.

106. Imperiali G, Meucci G, Alvisi C, et al. Segemental colitis associated with diverticula: a prospective study. Am J Gastroenterol 2000;95:1014–6.

107. Hawkey CJ. NSAIDs, Coxibs and the intestine. J Cardiovasc Pharmacol 2006;47:S72–5.

108. Faucheron J- L. Toxicity of non-steroidal anti-inflammatory drugs in the large bowel. Eur J Gastroenterol Hepatol 1999;11:389–92.

109. Rampton DS, McNeil NI, Sarner M. Analgesic ingestion and other factors preceding relapse in ulcerative colitis. Gut 1983;24:187–9.

110. Evanns JMM, McMahon AD, Murray FE, et al. Non-steroidal anti-inflammatory are associated with emergency admission to hospital for colitis due to inflammatory bowel disease. Gut 1997;40:619–22.

111. Felder JB, Korelitz BI, Rajapakse R, et al. Effect of NSAID drugs on inflammatory bowel disease: a case control study. Am J Gastroenterol 2000;85:1949–55.

112. Takeuchi K, Smale S, Puroshothaman P, et al. Prevalence and mechanism of non-steroidal anti-inflammatory drug-induced clinical relapse in patients with inflammatory bowel disease. Clin Gastroenterol Hepatol 2006;4:196–202.

113. Sandborn WJ, Stenson WF, Brynskov J, et al. Safety of celecoxib in patients with ulcerative colitis in remission: a randomized, placebo controlled pilot study. Clin Gastroenterol Hepatol 2006;4:203–11.

114. Bresailer RS, Sandler RS, Quan H, et al. Adenomatous Polyp Prevention on Vioxx Trial I. Cardiovascular events associated with rofecoxib in a colorectal adenoma chemoprevention trial. N Engl J Med 2005;352:1092–102.

115. Solomon SD, McMurray JJ, Pfeffer MA, et al. Adenoma prevention with Celecoxib Study I. Cardiovascular risk associated with celecoxib in a clinical trial for colorectal adenoma prevention. N Engl J Med 2005;352:1071–80.

116. Brophy JM. Cardiovascular risk associated with celecoxib. N Engl J Med 2005;352:2648–50.

117. Korotinski S, Katz A, Malnick DH. Chronic ischaemic bowel diseases in the aged—go with the flow. Age Ageing 2005;34:10–6.

118. Green BT, Tendler DA. Ischemic colitis: a clinical review. Southampt Med J 2005;98:217–22.

Chronic Constipation in the Elderly

Ernest P. Bouras, MD[a],*, Eric G. Tangalos, MD[b]

KEYWORDS

- Constipation • Pelvic floor dysfunction • Defecation disorder
- Elderly • Geriatric • Management

DEFINITIONS AND EPIDEMIOLOGY
Constipation

Constipation is variably defined, and its diagnosis is often arbitrary. Physicians tend to consider stool frequency (<3 defecations per week),[1] whereas patients more often consider straining, stool consistency, incomplete evacuation, and nonproductive urges to have a bowel movement.[2] A combination of objective (stool frequency, manual maneuvers needed for defecation) and subjective (straining, lumpy or hard stools, incomplete evacuation, sensation of anorectal obstruction) symptoms are used in the Rome III criteria for constipation.[3]

Although most studies suggest an adult prevalence for constipation of about 15%, estimates range from 2% to 27%,[2,4–7] with the variability largely explained by the definitions used and population sampled. Like the definitions used, patient perception of constipation is variable, and simply asking patients if they are constipated is unsatisfactory. Most epidemiologic studies demonstrate a higher prevalence of constipation and laxative use in the elderly,[7–16] particularly in the institutionalized; studies suggest a prevalence for constipation as high as 50%, with up to 74% of nursing home residents using daily laxatives.[17–19]

In addition to advanced age, risk factors for chronic constipation (CC) include female sex, nonwhite race, physical inactivity, low income and educational level, medications, dietary intake, and depression.[6–8,10–12,16,20–26] Severe constipation is seen almost exclusively in women, with elderly women having rates of constipation two to three times higher than that of their male counterparts.[7,8,10,16,27] The elderly, who often underestimate their stool frequency,[17] frequently plan their days around their bowel movements, and treatments often precipitate loose stools and incontinence.

Constipation ranks among the top five most common physician diagnoses for gastrointestinal disorders among outpatient clinic visits,[28] and the accompanying

---

[a] Department of Medicine, Division of Gastroenterology and Hepatology, E6A, Mayo Clinic, 4500 San Pablo Road, Jacksonville, FL 32224, USA
[b] Department of Medicine, Primary Care Internal Medicine, Mayo Clinic, 200 First Street SW, Rochester, MN 55906, USA
* Corresponding author.
E-mail address: bouras.ernest@mayo.edu (E.P. Bouras).

Gastroenterol Clin N Am 38 (2009) 463–480
doi:10.1016/j.gtc.2009.06.001
0889-8553/09/$ – see front matter © 2009 Elsevier Inc. All rights reserved.

use of health care resources is substantial.[29,30] A recent study identified more than 7 million physician visits per year for constipation in the United States,[31] the majority with primary care providers. However, this probably under-represents the true impact of constipation and subsequent medical use, as many people undoubtedly either do not seek medical attention or use over-the-counter remedies (either alone or in combination with those prescribed by their physician). Patients referred to gastroenterologists tend to represent more chronic or refractory cases.

Pelvic Floor Dysfunction

An appreciation of the contribution of the pelvic floor to defecation is essential in understanding constipation. The functional anatomy of the pelvic floor consists of the pelvic diaphragm (levator ani and coccygeus muscles) and anal sphincters, innervated by the sacral nerve roots (S_{2-4}) and pudendal nerve (**Fig. 1**). Normal functioning of this neuromuscular unit allows the efficient elimination of stool from the rectum. Although the exact prevalence of pelvic floor dysfunction (PFD) in constipation is unknown, studies in tertiary care centers have demonstrated a prevalence of 50% or more.[32,33] Common in the young, abnormalities of pelvic floor function are frequent in the elderly, especially in older women.[34-36]

PFD is more common in patients with a history of anorectal surgery or other pelvic floor trauma (including childbirth). In addition to defecatory dysfunction, PFD manifests with disorders of urinary and sexual function. As it relates to constipation, PFD may be more appropriately termed a functional defecation disorder (FDD), which can be characterized by (a) paradoxic contractions or inadequate relaxation of the pelvic floor muscles, or (b) inadequate propulsive forces during attempted defecation.[37]

PATHOPHYSIOLOGY

The major causes of constipation include slow colonic transit and PFD. Although the prevalence and clinical significance are unknown, complications of diverticular

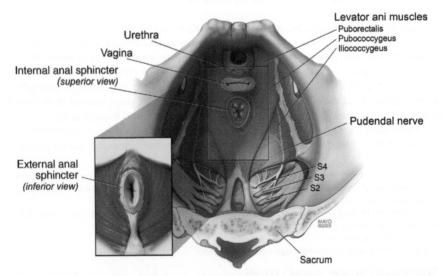

Fig. 1. Functional anatomy of the pelvic floor. *Courtesy of* the Mayo Clinic, Rochester, MN; with permission.

disease and ischemic colitis may rarely play a role in the elderly. A variety of psychosocial and behavioral issues are also important, and more than 1 mechanism may be present in a single patient. Patients in whom no cause is identified can be categorized as having normal transit constipation.

Aging Process

It is not surprising that the altered mechanical properties (eg, loss of plasticity and compliance), altered macroscopic structural changes (eg, diverticulosis), and altered control of the pelvic floor seen with advancing age impact bowel structure and function.[34] However, although the aging process inevitably generates changes in the colon, the full extent and physiologic impact of those changes on continence and defecatory function remain unclear. In addition, many therapeutic trials exclude older patients, further limiting our appreciation of colonic function and responsiveness in this age group. Indeed, the clinical picture is complicated by more than the aging process itself, as there are a multitude of additional factors ubiquitous amongst many of the aged that impact bowel function (List 1).

List 1: Ten D's of constipation in the elderly

- Drugs (side effects)
- Defecatory dysfunction
- Degenerative disease
- Decreased dietary intake
- Dementia
- Decreased mobility/activity
- Dependence on others for assistance
- Decreased privacy
- Dehydration
- Depression

Enteric Nervous System

The effect of age on the anatomy and function of the enteric nervous system (ENS) is incompletely understood. Although the analysis of changes in the neuronal number in the ENS is not straightforward, studies do suggest an age-related loss of colonic neurons[38–40] and changes in the morphology of the myenteric plexus of the human colon.[41] A recent study demonstrated the selective age-related loss of neurons that express choline acetyltransferase that was accompanied by sparing of neuronal nitric oxide expressing neurons in the human colon.[40] Theoretically, this could result in a progressive relative increase in inhibitory neurons with advancing age. However, little is known about the regional distribution of neurotransmitters, the impact of aging on the interstitial cells of Cajal, and the influence of the neuronal functional reserve as the colon ages.[34]

The factors that contribute to the presumed alteration in motility during aging are undoubtedly complex, with different effects in different regions of the gut.[42] The eventual effect of these factors on colonic function and defecation is unclear. Overall, gastrointestinal function seems to be well preserved with increasing age,[43] and most healthy elderly individuals have normal bowel function.[15]

Colonic Transit

Investigations differ with regard to the effect of aging on colonic transit; some studies have found a slowing in the elderly,[44,45] whereas others have detected no significant difference between the elderly and their younger counterparts.[46–49] Whereas some believe that the normal process of aging reduces the propulsive efficacy of the colon,[50] it is less clear whether this may be related to qualitative or quantitative differences in the colon and ENS, or the numerous causes of secondarily slowed colonic transit that are common amongst the elderly (see **Table 1**). Primary or idiopathic slow colonic transit and global gastrointestinal motility disturbances (intestinal pseudo-obstruction) are uncommon, and few patients have primary colonic inertia or megacolon.[51] Typically, there are straightforward explanations for slow transit, such as the often overlooked but modifiable causes of medication effects and PFD with secondary slowing of colonic transit by inhibitory reflexes.

Pelvic Floor Function

Normal defecation is accomplished through a series of coordinated, neurologically mediated movements of the pelvic floor and anal sphincter (**Fig. 2**). Abnormalities in this complex series of actions lead to abnormal stool expulsion, or a functional outlet obstruction to defecation.[52,53] This may be secondary inadequate relaxation or paradoxical contraction of the musculature or the inability to produce the effective propulsive forces needed to expel the stool.

Whereas some studies show no differences in anorectal function between the elderly and their younger counterparts,[54,55] other physiologic studies have demonstrated various abnormalities with advancing age, including decreased rectal

Table 1
Common associations with constipation in the elderly

Nongastrointestinal Medical Conditions	Medications
Endocrine and metabolic disorders	• Analgesics (opiates, tramadol, NSAIDs)
• Diabetes mellitus	• Anticholinergic agents
• Hypothyroidsim	• Calcium channel blockers
• Hyperparathyroidism	• Tricyclic antidepressants
• Chronic renal disease	• Anti-parkinsonian drugs (dopaminergic agents)
Electrolyte disturbances	• Antacids (calcium and aluminum)
• Hypercalcemia	• Calcium supplements
• Hypokalemia	• Bile acid binders
• Hypermagnesemia	• Iron supplements
Neurologic disorders	• Antihistamines
• Parkinson disease	• Diuretics (furosemide, hydrochlorothiazide)
• Multiple sclerosis	• Iron supplements
• Autonomic neuropathy	• Antipsychotics (phenothiazine derivatives)
• Spinal cord lesions	• Anticonvulsants
• Dementia	
Myopathic disorders	
• Amyloidosis	
• Scleroderma	
Other	
• Depression	
• General disability	

Abbreviation: NSAIDs, nonsteroidal anti-inflammatory drugs.

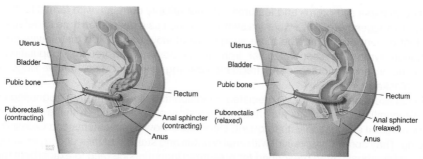

Fig. 2. Dynamics of defecation. At rest (*left panel*), the puborectalis sling holds the rectum at an angle and the anal sphincters are closed. On normal defecation (*right panel*), (a) the puborectalis relaxes, (b) the anorectal angle straightens, (c) the pelvic floor descends, and (d) the anal sphincter relaxes, allowing stool expulsion when accompanied by adequate propulsive force. *Courtesy of* the Mayo Clinic, Rochester, MN; with permission.

compliance, increased urge thresholds for defecation, and decreased rest and squeeze pressures in the anal canal.[34–36,56–59] PFD is a comprehensive phrase, and other terms relating to defecatory dysfunction include dyssynergia, anismus, obstructed defecation, outlet delay, among others. Although there are subtle differences to the meanings, the key concept of disordered defecation secondary to abnormal pelvic floor function is the same.

In addition to the physiologic types of PFD, specific anatomic abnormalities (rectoceles, sigmoidoceles, rectoanal intussusception, and so forth) may impact defecation. Like the pelvic floor laxity that often accompanies these anatomic findings, they are common in elderly women, but the significance is not always clear. Along with the usual factors associated with aging and constipation, appreciating the pelvic floor and its function is essential for effectual patient management.

Psychosocial and Behavioral Factors

In addition to the personality factors, psychological distress, and a history of physical or sexual abuse that have been associated with constipation,[23,24,60–63] the elderly are at risk secondary to decreased mobility, altered dietary intake, dependency on others, and issues that may develop from social isolation. PFD is a type of behavioral disorder that may be learned at any age in response to specific demands or physical or mental injury. The elderly may ignore calls to defecate, leading to fecal retention. Chronic retention can lead to suppression of rectal sensation, which decreases the desire to defecate. Ultimately, only large stool volumes may be perceived, and, consequently, there is difficulty with rectal evacuation.[64] Defecation disorders interfere with quality of life[65–69] and may alter interpersonal, intimate, and interfamily relationships.

CLINICAL PRESENTATION

As with the definition of constipation, there is variability in patient presentation. Excessive or prolonged straining, assisting stool evacuation by assuming certain positions or with rectal or vaginal digital manipulation, and the sensation of incomplete rectal evacuation are among several features that suggest PFD.[68,70] Others include urinary and sexual dysfunction, previous pelvic or rectal surgery, history of anal fissures, prolapse, and a history of pelvic floor trauma, including child birthing.

Although these symptoms and features may not reliably correlate with formal testing, they are suggestive of PFD, whereas symptoms such as a decreased urge to defecate and infrequent stools may be more suggestive of slow transit.[71] In the elderly, constipation symptoms seem to differ from those observed in younger populations, with the elderly reporting more frequent straining, self-digitation, and feelings of anal blockage.[8,72,73]

Fecal seepage is an underappreciated condition that is frequently misdiagnosed as fecal incontinence.[74,75] Patients often have a history of constipation with the sensation of poor rectal evacuation with frequent, incomplete bowel movements and excessive wiping. They commonly present with anal pruritus and staining of their undergarments. The antidiarrheals often prescribed for presumed incontinence tend to exacerbate the situation. Fecal impaction and overflow incontinence may be associated findings, particularly in the infirmed. Paradoxically, the problem is one of obstructed defecation than true incontinence. A thorough history and examination are essential, especially in those with altered cognitive function.

In addition to fecal seepage and incontinence, fecal impaction can lead to stercoral ulceration and bleeding. CC may be associated with pelvic floor laxity and accompanying rectal prolapse in addition to urinary and sexual dysfunction. Suppression of defecation has been shown to slow gastric emptying[76] and right colon transit,[77] and patients with CC have been shown to have prolonged mouth-to-cecum transit time.[78] It follows that reflex slowing of more proximal gut function can precipitate symptoms. Indeed, constipated patients do have an increase in dyspepsia, abdominal cramping, bloating, flatulence, heartburn, nausea, and vomiting.[10,22,79,80]

Other features to look for include the use of constipating medications, a general decline in physical or mental health, coexisting medical conditions, dietary habits and general psychosocial situation. Chronic pain, which is common in institutionalized patients, often leads to the use of constipating analgesics, which should be assessed. The presence of alarm features, such as rectal bleeding and weight loss, and a family or personal history of colon cancer should be ascertained.

DIAGNOSTIC APPROACH

Most patients will present to their primary care physician for the initial evaluation and management of constipation. Rather than focusing on set criteria, it is important to establish the patient's understanding and characterization of what constipation means to them. Various strategies for the initial diagnosis and treatment of constipation have been employed. Although there is limited data to support their routine use, standard diagnostic studies typically include baseline blood work and structural tests to exclude any significant metabolic or anatomic abnormalities.

Patients with persistent constipation, normal investigations, and a failed response to initial empiric therapies are the ones typically referred to the gastroenterologist. A stepwise, individualized approach to patients with CC is useful. Pursuing relevant studies that help categorize patients as to the cause of their constipation facilitates selection of the appropriate therapy for each specific physiologic subgroup.[70,81]

History and Physical Examination

A comprehensive history, carefully assessing relevant clinical features, including a thorough medication review, is needed. The physical examination is not complete without a thorough perianal and digital rectal examination, which goes beyond looking for mass lesions, anal strictures, fissures, or stool impaction (**Fig. 3**).[82]

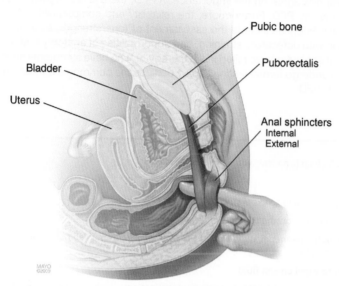

Pubic bone

Puborectalis

Bladder

Uterus

Anal sphincters
Internal
External

Fig. 3. Anorectal examination. With the patient in the left lateral position, the examiner should assess: (*a*) resting sphincter tone and presence of spasm, (*b*) sensation, including the presence of pain, (*c*) the ability to squeeze, and (*d*) coordination of the pelvic floor and rectal muscles and extent of perineal descent during simulated defecatory straining (expelling the examiner's finger). *Courtesy of* the Mayo Clinic, Rochester, MN; with permission.

Metabolic and Structural Evaluation

Assessing the complete blood count, electrolyte balance, calcium homeostasis and thyroid function are common, but these investigations rarely identify the cause of CC. The yield of colonoscopy and barium enema in patients with constipation is the same as the general population;[83,84] however, diagnostic studies are indicated in patients with alarm symptoms (eg, hematochezia, weight loss) and for the acute onset of constipation in the elderly. Routine colon cancer screening is recommended for all patients 50 years or older. Plain abdominal radiographs can assess fecal load, impaction, or obstruction.

Colonic Transit

Radiopaque marker studies are an inexpensive and widely available way to assess colon transit.[48,85] Patients should maintain a high fiber diet and abstain from medicines used to treat constipation. In addition to total marker counts, marker distribution may also be helpful, as proximal retention suggests colonic dysfunction, whereas the retention of markers exclusively in the lower left colon is more suggestive of a defecatory disorder. Scintigraphic techniques allow for shorter studies (24–48 hours) and decreased radiation exposure.[86] PFD, medications, diet, and the presence of excessive stool or impaction affect transit. Some advocate bowel cleansing before a transit assessment, which could be considered if severe, persistent constipation is unresponsive to multiple therapies, if PFD has been excluded, and if surgical treatment is being considered as an option.

Pelvic Floor Function

Although experts agree on the importance of PFD, there is less agreement on which tests best identify PFD. Furthermore, the reliability and comparability of many tests are unknown. Priorities include the assessment of tone/strength, sensation, control/coordination with defecatory straining, and abnormalities of anatomy that may impact function. Patients who have failed initial therapy or who have symptoms suggestive of PFD should undergo formal testing. **Box 1** outlines the common diagnostic findings in patients with PFD.

Box 1
Diagnostic findings in patients with defecatory disorders

History

- Prolonged straining to expel stool
- Unusual postures on the toilet to facilitate stool expulsion
- Support of the perineum, digitation of the rectum, or posterior vaginal pressure to facilitate rectal emptying
- Inability to expel enema fluid
- Constipation after subtotal colectomy for constipation

Rectal examination (with patient in left lateral position)

Inspection

- Anus pulled forward while the patient is bearing down
- Anal verge descends less than 1.0 or greater than 3.5 cm (or beyond the ischial tuberosities) while the patient is bearing down
- Perineum balloons down while the patient is bearing down, and rectal mucosa partially prolapses through the anal canal

Palpation

- High anal sphincter tone at rest
- Anal sphincter pressure during voluntary contraction is only slightly higher than tone at rest
- Perineum and examining finger descend less than 1.0 or greater than 3.5 cm while patient simulates straining during defecation
- Puborectalis muscle is tender on palpation through the rectal wall posteriorly, or palpation produces pain
- Palpable mucosal prolapse during straining
- Defect in anterior wall of the rectum, suggestive of a rectocele

Anorectal manometry and balloon expulsion (with patient in left lateral position)

- Average tone of anal sphincter at rest of greater than 80 mm Hg (or >60 cm water)
- Average pressure of anal sphincter during contraction of greater than 180 mm Hg (or >240 cm water)
- Failure to expel balloon

(*From* Lembo A, Camilleri M. Chronic constipation. N Engl J Med 2003;349(14):1360–8; with permission.)

Anorectal manometry with balloon expulsion testing provides measurements that relay key information about the motor and sensory control of the anorectum and pelvic floor.[87–90] Simulated defecation allows assessment of synergy and propulsive force. Evacuation proctography (defecography) attempts to identify any anatomic or functional abnormalities that may contribute to outlet obstruction. Various techniques may be used (eg, barium defecography, dynamic magnetic resonance imaging) depending on local expertise.[91–94] The goal is to assess the control of the dynamics of defecation and the ability of the patient to empty the rectum. Caution must be used, as the clinical significance of various anatomic abnormalities is often unclear. Rectoceles are common but may be considered clinically significant if they fill preferentially or fail to empty during simulated defecation.

TREATMENT SUGGESTIONS

Treatment of CC depends on the underlying physiologic cause, being mindful of other factors that may influence the presentation (eg, ten D's of constipation). As a general rule, patients who do not respond to fiber supplementation can be advanced to osmotic laxatives, which can be titrated to clinical response. Stimulant laxatives and prokinetic agents are typically reserved for patients with more refractory constipation. Throughout any treatment program, one should remain vigilant of PFD, as pelvic floor rehabilitation is the treatment of choice. Surgery is rarely indicated for constipation, exclusion of PFD is essential, and outcomes in the elderly are uncertain. Fecal impaction should be cleared before instituting maintenance regimens.

No single agent or program is best for all patients or situations. Treatment needs to be tailored not only to the cause, but to medical history, medications, overall clinical status, mental and physical abilities, tolerance to various agents, and realistic treatment prospects. Monitoring bowel movement frequency, stooling patterns, fecal soiling, and use of laxatives may help in the development of an overall treatment regimen tailored to the individual patient. Specific issues for institutionalized patients need to be addressed with standardized, supervised bowel programs. The following brief treatment overview highlights some general overall comments regarding various agents and approaches.

Bulking Agents

Carefully increasing fiber intake from 15 to 25 g/d may be accomplished with dietary adjustments, and supplements (**Table 2**). Although increasing water intake on its own has not been shown to improve constipation, maintaining adequate fluid intake is prudent with fiber supplementation to avoid excessive bulk, which may exacerbate CC. A well-formed, softer stool that is easier to pass is the ultimate goal. Fluid intake

Table 2 Commonly used laxative agents		
Bulk-Forming	**Osmotic**	**Stimulant**
Psyllium (ispaghula)	Saline laxatives	Anthraquinones
Bran	• Magnesium salts	• Senna
Methylcellulose	Poorly absorbed sugars	Diphenylmethane derivatives
Calcium polycarbophil	• Sorbitol	• Bisacodyl
	• Lactulose	
	Polyethylene glycol	

needs to be monitored in patients with cardiac or renal disease, and the need to maintain adequate hydration may be a limitation for some.

Although there is little to no relationship between dietary fiber intake and whole gut transit time,[95] empiric fiber supplementation is a common and reasonable first step in the management of CC. Increasing the dose of fiber carefully over several weeks to a month may lessen common side effects (bloating, gas, and distention) and enhance compliance. Synthetic supplements are often tolerated better than others. Patients with severely delayed colonic transit respond poorly to dietary fiber.[95,96] Trials looking at bulking agents are of suboptimal design and most are plagued by small sample sizes and short study duration.[27,97]

Laxatives

Osmotic laxatives work by retaining or drawing water into the gut lumen and are a reasonable choice for patients not responding to fiber supplementation (see **Table 2**). As there is no clearly superior osmotic agent, the laxative should be based on relevant medical history (cardiac or renal status), possible drug interactions, cost, and side effects. The dose should be titrated to the clinical response. For chronic or more severe constipation, regular dosing is indicated. Per FDA-approved prescribing information, high doses of polyethylene glycol may produce excessive stool frequency, especially in elderly nursing home residents, and nausea, abdominal bloating, cramping, and flatulence may occur.[27] Many patients rely on the laxative action of prune juice as part of their daily regimen, or intermittently, to modify bowel function.

Contrary to the widely held belief, stimulant laxatives, which promote intestinal motility, do not seem to lead to bowel injury.[98,99] However, these drugs are better reserved for those with a failed response to osmotic agents, and may be required in the management of opioid-induced constipation. Effective for many patients, studies with laxatives in the elderly are limited and are of suboptimal design.[100] In general, the available data suggests minimal benefit with these agents.[27] Abdominal discomfort, electrolyte imbalances, allergic reactions and hepatotoxicity have been reported.[101] No recommendation as to any specific laxative class or single agent can be made with confidence.

Stool Softeners, Suppositories and Enemas

Useful for some, stool softeners are of limited overall efficacy.[97,102] Suppositories (eg, glycerin) help initiate or facilitate rectal evacuation. They may be used alone, in conjunction with meals (to capture the gastrocolic reflex), or in conjunction with other agents.[103] Suppositories, which usually work within minutes, may be tried as part of a behavioral program for those with obstructed defecation and in the institutionalized. In general, enemas may be used judiciously on an as-needed basis, particularly for obstructed defecation and to avoid fecal impaction. Routine use is typically discouraged but may be necessary. Whereas tap water enemas seem safe for more regular use, electrolyte imbalances are more common with phosphate enemas. Soapsuds enemas can cause rectal mucosal damage and are not recommended.

Prokinetics and Other Agents

Prokinetic agents are currently of limited availability. Cisapride has been removed from the market. Metoclopramide and erythromycin are of no obvious benefit in constipation. Found effective for CC in men and women younger than 65 years,[104,105] tegaserod, a serotonin (5-HT$_4$) receptor agonist, has not been tested specifically in the elderly. Although the drug seems effective in the management of constipation, use has been markedly restricted secondary to the risk of cardiac events. Prucalopride, a serotoninergic agent similar to tegaserod, accelerates colonic transit in patients with constipation,[106] and therapeutic trials have demonstrated efficacy for severe constipation.[107,108] Studies in the elderly are lacking, and the drug is not available in the United States.

Lubiprostone, a bicyclic fatty acid that activates chloride channels on the apical membrane of the intestinal epithelial cells, helps in constipation by moving water into the gut lumen.[109] In light of the cost, this medication is best reserved for a lack of efficacy of less expensive alternatives. The indications for this line of therapy in patients with a primary problem of PFD are not established.

Pelvic Floor Rehabilitation (Biofeedback)

Pelvic floor rehabilitation is the treatment of choice for PFD. Therapy focuses on sensory and muscular retraining of the rectum and pelvic floor, with the goals of normalization of sensation, muscular relaxation or strengthening, and improved defecatory dynamics with resolution of any paradoxical pelvic floor contractions. There are no obvious adverse effects of treatment. However, different therapeutic protocols exist, and the best approach is unclear.

Uncontrolled studies suggest that biofeedback is effective in more than 70% of patients,[110] and these findings have been confirmed in several randomized, controlled trials.[111–113] The presence of descending perineum syndrome may limit results.[114] Biofeedback has been shown to be superior to laxatives in patients with a FDD, and the effect was durable.[111] The key is identifying the problem and available therapeutic resources.

A patient's physical and mental abilities must be assessed. Although no physiologic, anatomic or demographic variables clearly impact treatment outcome, many believe that psychopathology may play a role.[62,110] Concomitant slow colon transit frequently requires simultaneous treatment. The efficacy of biofeedback in the elderly is unclear, and a realistic appraisal of the patient's physical and mental capabilities is necessary to assess the potential usefulness of this line of therapy.

Surgery

Although rarely indicated, subtotal colectomy with ileorectal anastomosis is the treatment of choice for medically refractory slow transit constipation but only if PFD is excluded.[115–117] Outcomes in the elderly are uncertain. Complications include diarrhea, incontinence, and bowel obstruction.[118] Extra caution should be used in patients with abdominal pain, which tends to respond poorly. Results of segmental colonic resections for constipation are disappointing.[119]

Surgical indications for PFD are poorly defined, and surgery should be considered only if functional significance can be determined.[117,119] Division of the puborectalis is not recommended.[120] Anatomic abnormalities (eg, rectoceles) are common but they are frequently the result of PFD. Treatment of the underlying PFD first is a reasonable treatment approach, with surgery reserved for those not responding to more conservative therapy.

Additional Comments

Adjunctive therapy may be necessary for psychopathology associated with CC, and maintaining adequate caloric intake is essential. Evidence does not support the popular notion that toxins from constipation harm the body or that irrigation is needed. There is no obvious significance of an elongated colon (dolichocolon), and surgical shortening does not lead to reliable clinical improvement.[99] Likewise, physical activity and water intake are controversial subjects, with unclear associations with colon transit and constipation.[99] There is no value in over hydrating a patient; families, long-term care facilities, and physicians should just guard against dehydration.

Although mineral oil, colchicine[121] and misoprostol[122,123] may improve constipation, these agents have potential side effects and complications that likely outweigh any potential benefits. Their use in the elderly has not been explored. Emerging therapies, such as sacral nerve stimulation, botulinum toxin injection for PFD, alteration of the bacterial milieu, and several novel medications may play more of a role in the future management of CC.

SUMMARY

CC in the elderly is common, is variably defined, has a significant impact on quality of life and the use of health care resources. A careful history, medication assessment, and physical examination are helpful in obtaining relevant clues that help direct management. Physiologic categorization of the cause leading to patient presentation improves management outcomes, realizing that many causes can be present in one patient, and many factors influence the clinical presentation of an older patient. Fiber supplementation and osmotic laxatives are effective for many patients CC. A consistent history or inadequate response to standard initial therapy should prompt an assessment for PFD. If identified, and the patient is a reasonable treatment candidate, pelvic floor rehabilitation (biofeedback) is the treatment of choice. Surgery is rarely indicated in CC. Special effort should be taken to identify features inherent to the elderly, and treatment should be based on the patient's overall clinical status and capabilities.

REFERENCES

1. Drossman DA, Sandler RS, McKee DC, et al. Bowel patterns among subjects not seeking health care. Use of a questionnaire to identify a population with bowel dysfunction. Gastroenterology 1982;83(3):529–34.
2. Pare P, Ferrazzi S, Thompson WG, et al. An epidemiological survey of constipation in Canada: definitions, rates, demographics, and predictors of health care seeking. Am J Gastroenterol 2001;96(11):3130–7.
3. Longstreth GF. Functional bowel disorders: functional constipation. In: Drossman DA, editor. The functional gastrointestinal disorders. 3rd edition. Lawrence (KS): Allen Press, Inc.; 2006. p. 515–23.
4. Stewart WF, Liberman JN, Sandler RS, et al. Epidemiology of constipation (EPOC) study in the United States: relation of clinical subtypes to sociodemographic features. Am J Gastroenterol 1999;94(12):3530–40.
5. Sonnenberg A, Koch TR. Physician visits in the United States for constipation: 1958 to 1986. Dig Dis Sci 1989;34(4):606–11.
6. Higgins PD, Johanson JF. Epidemiology of constipation in North America: a systematic review. Am J Gastroenterol 2004;99(4):750–9.
7. Johanson JF, Sonnenberg A, Koch TR. Clinical epidemiology of chronic constipation. J Clin Gastroenterol 1989;11(5):525–36.
8. Talley NJ, Fleming KC, Evans JM, et al. Constipation in an elderly community: a study of prevalence and potential risk factors. Am J Gastroenterol 1996; 91(1):19–25.
9. Crane SJ, Talley NJ. Chronic gastrointestinal symptoms in the elderly. Clin Geriatr Med 2007;23(4):721–34, v.

10. Wald A, Scarpignato C, Mueller-Lissner S, et al. A multinational survey of prevalence and patterns of laxative use among adults with self-defined constipation. Aliment Pharmacol Ther 2008;28(7):917–30.

11. Sandler RS, Jordan MC, Shelton BJ. Demographic and dietary determinants of constipation in the US population. Am J Public Health 1990;80(2):185–9.

12. Everhart JE, Go VL, Johannes RS, et al. A longitudinal survey of self-reported bowel habits in the United States. Dig Dis Sci 1989;34(8):1153–62.

13. Whitehead WE, Drinkwater D, Cheskin LJ, et al. Constipation in the elderly living at home. Definition, prevalence, and relationship to lifestyle and health status. J Am Geriatr Soc 1989;37(5):423–9.

14. Donald IP, Smith RG, Cruikshank JG, et al. A study of constipation in the elderly living at home. Gerontology 1985;31(2):112–8.

15. Harari D, Gurwitz JH, Avorn J, et al. Bowel habit in relation to age and gender. Findings from the National Health Interview Survey and clinical implications. Arch Intern Med 1996;156(3):315–20.

16. Choung RS, Locke GR 3rd, Schleck CD, et al. Cumulative incidence of chronic constipation: a population-based study 1988–2003. Aliment Pharmacol Ther 2007;26(11–12):1521–8.

17. Harari D, Gurwitz JH, Avorn J, et al. Constipation: assessment and management in an institutionalized elderly population. J Am Geriatr Soc 1994;42(9):947–52.

18. Talley NJ. Definitions, epidemiology, and impact of chronic constipation. Rev Gastroenterol Disord 2004;4(Suppl 2):S3–10.

19. Primrose WR, Capewell AE, Simpson GK, et al. Prescribing patterns observed in registered nursing homes and long-stay geriatric wards. Age Ageing 1987;16(1):25–8.

20. Sonnenberg A, Koch TR. Epidemiology of constipation in the United States. Dis Colon Rectum 1989;32(1):1–8.

21. Connell AM, Hilton C, Irvine G, et al. Variation of bowel habit in two population samples. Br Med J 1965;2(5470):1095–9.

22. Drossman DA, Li Z, Andruzzi E, et al. U.S. householder survey of functional gastrointestinal disorders. Prevalence, sociodemography, and health impact. Dig Dis Sci 1993;38(9):1569–80.

23. Merkel IS, Locher J, Burgio K, et al. Physiologic and psychologic characteristics of an elderly population with chronic constipation. Am J Gastroenterol 1993;88(11):1854–9.

24. Towers AL, Burgio KL, Locher JL, et al. Constipation in the elderly: influence of dietary, psychological, and physiological factors. J Am Geriatr Soc 1994;42(7):701–6.

25. Talley NJ, Jones M, Nuyts G, et al. Risk factors for chronic constipation based on a general practice sample. Am J Gastroenterol 2003;98(5):1107–11.

26. Dukas L, Willett WC, Giovannucci EL. Association between physical activity, fiber intake, and other lifestyle variables and constipation in a study of women. Am J Gastroenterol 2003;98(8):1790–6.

27. Brandt LJ, Prather CM, Quigley EM, et al. Systematic review on the management of chronic constipation in North America. Am J Gastroenterol 2005;100(Suppl 1):S5–21.

28. Shaheen NJ, Hansen RA, Morgan DR, et al. The burden of gastrointestinal and liver diseases, 2006. Am J Gastroenterol 2006;101(9):2128–38.

29. Martin BC, Barghout V, Cerulli A. Direct medical costs of constipation in the United States. Manag Care Interface 2006;19(12):43–9.

30. Dennison C, Prasad M, Lloyd A, et al. The health-related quality of life and economic burden of constipation. Pharmacoeconomics 2005;23(5):461–76.
31. Shah ND, Chitkara DK, Locke GR, et al. Ambulatory care for constipation in the United States, 1993–2004. Am J Gastroenterol 2008;103(7):1746–53.
32. Surrenti E, Rath DM, Pemberton JH, et al. Audit of constipation in a tertiary referral gastroenterology practice. Am J Gastroenterol 1995;90(9):1471–5.
33. Kuijpers HC. Application of the colorectal laboratory in diagnosis and treatment of functional constipation. Dis Colon Rectum 1990;33(1):35–9.
34. Camilleri M, Lee JS, Viramontes B, et al. Insights into the pathophysiology and mechanisms of constipation, irritable bowel syndrome, and diverticulosis in older people. J Am Geriatr Soc 2000;48(9):1142–50.
35. Bannister JJ, Abouzekry L, Read NW. Effect of aging on anorectal function. Gut 1987;28(3):353–7.
36. Laurberg S, Swash M. Effects of aging on the anorectal sphincters and their innervation. Dis Colon Rectum 1989;32(9):737–42.
37. Wald A, Bharucha A, Enck P, et al. Functional anorectal disorders: functional defecation disorders. In: Drossman DA, editor. The functional gastrointestinal disorders. 3rd edition. Lawrence (KS): Allen Press, Inc.; 2006. p. 663–75.
38. Gomes OA, de Souza RR, Liberti EA. A preliminary investigation of the effects of aging on the nerve cell number in the myenteric ganglia of the human colon. Gerontology 1997;43(4):210–7.
39. Phillips RJ, Powley TL. Innervation of the gastrointestinal tract: patterns of aging. Auton Neurosci 2007;136(1–2):1–19.
40. Bernard CE, Gibbons SJ, Gomez-Pinilla PJ, et al. Effect of age on the enteric nervous system of the human colon. Neurogastroenterol Motil 2009;21:746–53.
41. Hanani M, Fellig Y, Udassin R, et al. Age-related changes in the morphology of the myenteric plexus of the human colon. Auton Neurosci 2004;113(1–2):71–8.
42. Saffrey MJ. Ageing of the enteric nervous system. Mech Ageing Dev 2004; 125(12):899–906.
43. Hall K, Wiley JW. Age associated changes in gastrointestinal function. In: Hazzard JP, Blass WR, Ettinger WH, et al, editors. Principles of geriatric medicine and gerontology. 4th edition. New York: McGraw-Hill; 1999. p. 835–42.
44. Melkersson M, Andersson H, Bosaeus I, et al. Intestinal transit time in constipated and non-constipated geriatric patients. Scand J Gastroenterol 1983; 18(5):593–7.
45. Madsen JL, Graff J. Effects of ageing on gastrointestinal motor function. Age Ageing 2004;33(2):154–9.
46. Evans JM, Fleming KC, Talley NJ, et al. Relation of colonic transit to functional bowel disease in older people: a population-based study. J Am Geriatr Soc 1998;46(1):83–7.
47. Meir R, Beglinger C, Dederding J, et al. Influence of age, gender, hormonal status and smoking habits on colonic transit time. Neurogastroenterol Motil 1995;7:235–8.
48. Metcalf AM, Phillips SF, Zinsmeister AR, et al. Simplified assessment of segmental colonic transit. Gastroenterology 1987;92(1):40–7.
49. Eastwood HD. Bowel transit studies in the elderly: radio-opaque markers in the investigation of constipation. Gerontol Clin (Basel) 1972;14(3):154–9.
50. Salles N. Basic mechanisms of the aging gastrointestinal tract. Dig Dis 2007; 25(2):112–7.
51. Gattuso JM, Kamm MA. Clinical features of idiopathic megarectum and idiopathic megacolon. Gut 1997;41(1):93–9.

52. Rao SS, Welcher KD, Leistikow JS. Obstructive defecation: a failure of rectoanal coordination. Am J Gastroenterol 1998;93(7):1042–50.
53. Rao SS. Dyssynergic defecation. Gastroenterol Clin North Am 2001;30(1):97–114.
54. Loening-Baucke V, Anuras S. Anorectal manometry in healthy elderly subjects. J Am Geriatr Soc 1984;32(9):636–9.
55. Loening-Baucke V, Anuras S. Effects of age and sex on anorectal manometry. Am J Gastroenterol 1985;80(1):50–3.
56. McHugh SM, Diamant NE. Effect of age, gender, and parity on anal canal pressures. Contribution of impaired anal sphincter function to fecal incontinence. Dig Dis Sci 1987;32(7):726–36.
57. Akervall S, Nordgren S, Fasth S, et al. The effects of age, gender, and parity on rectoanal functions in adults. Scand J Gastroenterol 1990;25(12):1247–56.
58. Orr WC, Chen CL. Aging and neural control of the GI tract: IV. Clinical and physiological aspects of gastrointestinal motility and aging. Am J Physiol Gastrointest Liver Physiol 2002;283(6):G1226–31.
59. Enck P, Kuhlbusch R, Lubke H, et al. Age and sex and anorectal manometry in incontinence. Dis Colon Rectum 1989;32(12):1026–30.
60. Wald A, Hinds JP, Caruana BJ. Psychological and physiological characteristics of patients with severe idiopathic constipation. Gastroenterology 1989;97(4):932–7.
61. Leroi AM, Bernier C, Watier A, et al. Prevalence of sexual abuse among patients with functional disorders of the lower gastrointestinal tract. Int J Colorectal Dis 1995;10(4):200–6.
62. Nehra V, Bruce BK, Rath-Harvey DM, et al. Psychological disorders in patients with evacuation disorders and constipation in a tertiary practice. Am J Gastroenterol 2000;95(7):1755–8.
63. Grotz RL, Pemberton JH, Talley NJ, et al. Discriminant value of psychological distress, symptom profiles, and segmental colonic dysfunction in outpatients with severe idiopathic constipation. Gut 1994;35(6):798–802.
64. Talley NJ, O'Keefe EA, Zinsmeister AR, et al. Prevalence of gastrointestinal symptoms in the elderly: a population-based study. Gastroenterology 1992;102(3):895–901.
65. Irvine EJ, Ferrazzi S, Pare P, et al. Health-related quality of life in functional GI disorders: focus on constipation and resource utilization. Am J Gastroenterol 2002;97(8):1986–93.
66. O'Keefe EA, Talley NJ, Zinsmeister AR, et al. Bowel disorders impair functional status and quality of life in the elderly: a population-based study. J Gerontol A Biol Sci Med Sci 1995;50(4):M184–9.
67. Wolfsen CR, Barker JC, Mitteness LS. Constipation in the daily lives of frail elderly people. Arch Fam Med 1993;2(8):853–8.
68. Rao SS, Tuteja AK, Vellema T, et al. Dyssynergic defecation: demographics, symptoms, stool patterns, and quality of life. J Clin Gastroenterol 2004;38(8):680–5.
69. Glia A, Lindberg G. Quality of life in patients with different types of functional constipation. Scand J Gastroenterol 1997;32(11):1083–9.
70. Lembo A, Camilleri M. Chronic constipation. N Engl J Med 2003;349(14):1360–8.
71. Mertz H, Naliboff B, Mayer EA. Symptoms and physiology in severe chronic constipation. Am J Gastroenterol 1999;94(1):131–8.
72. Talley NJ, Weaver AL, Zinsmeister AR, et al. Functional constipation and outlet delay: a population-based study. Gastroenterology 1993;105(3):781–90.

73. Harari D, Gurwitz JH, Avorn J, et al. How do older persons define constipation? Implications for therapeutic management. J Gen Intern Med 1997;12(1):63–6.

74. Rao SS. Diagnosis and management of fecal incontinence. American College of Gastroenterology Practice Parameters Committee. Am J Gastroenterol 2004; 99(8):1585–604.

75. Rao SS, Ozturk R, Stessman M. Investigation of the pathophysiology of fecal seepage. Am J Gastroenterol 2004;99(11):2204–9.

76. Tjeerdsma HC, Smout AJ, Akkermans LM. Voluntary suppression of defecation delays gastric emptying. Dig Dis Sci 1993;38(5):832–6.

77. Klauser AG, Voderholzer WA, Heinrich CA, et al. Behavioral modification of colonic function. Can constipation be learned? Dig Dis Sci 1990;35(10):1271–5.

78. Marzio L, Del Bianco R, Donne MD, et al. Mouth-to-cecum transit time in patients affected by chronic constipation: effect of glucomannan. Am J Gastroenterol 1989;84(8):888–91.

79. Talley NJ, Dennis EH, Schettler-Duncan VA, et al. Overlapping upper and lower gastrointestinal symptoms in irritable bowel syndrome patients with constipation or diarrhea. Am J Gastroenterol 2003;98(11):2454–9.

80. Locke GR 3rd, Zinsmeister AR, Fett SL, et al. Overlap of gastrointestinal symptom complexes in a US community. Neurogastroenterol Motil 2005;17(1):29–34.

81. Locke GR 3rd, Pemberton JH, Phillips SF. AGA technical review on constipation. American Gastroenterological Association. Gastroenterology 2000;119(6): 1766–78.

82. Talley NJ. How to do and interpret a rectal examination in gastroenterology. Am J Gastroenterol 2008;103(4):820–2.

83. Pepin C, Ladabaum U. The yield of lower endoscopy in patients with constipation: survey of a university hospital, a public county hospital, and a Veterans Administration medical center. Gastrointest Endosc 2002;56(3):325–32.

84. Patriquin H, Martelli H, Devroede G. Barium enema in chronic constipation: is it meaningful? Gastroenterology 1978;75(4):619–22.

85. Hinton JM, Lennard-Jones JE, Young AC. A new method for studying gut transit times using radioopaque markers. Gut 1969;10(10):842–7.

86. Stivland T, Camilleri M, Vassallo M, et al. Scintigraphic measurement of regional gut transit in idiopathic constipation. Gastroenterology 1991;101(1):107–15.

87. Diamant NE, Kamm MA, Wald A, et al. AGA technical review on anorectal testing techniques. Gastroenterology 1999;116(3):735–60.

88. Preston DM, Lennard-Jones JE. Anismus in chronic constipation. Dig Dis Sci 1985;30(5):413–8.

89. Fleshman JW, Dreznik Z, Cohen E, et al. Balloon expulsion test facilitates diagnosis of pelvic floor outlet obstruction due to nonrelaxing puborectalis muscle. Dis Colon Rectum 1992;35(11):1019–25.

90. Rao SS, Ozturk R, Laine L. Clinical utility of diagnostic tests for constipation in adults: a systematic review. Am J Gastroenterol 2005;100(7):1605–15.

91. Bharucha AE, Fletcher JG, Seide B, et al. Phenotypic variation in functional disorders of defecation. Gastroenterology 2005;128(5):1199–210.

92. Shorvon P, Marshall M. Evacuation proctography. In: Wexner SD, Zbar AP, Pescatori M, editors. Complex anorectal disorders investigation and management. New York: Springer; 2005. p. 171–98.

93. Mortele KJ, Fairhurst J. Dynamic MR defecography of the posterior compartment: indications, techniques and MRI features. Eur J Radiol 2007;61(3):462–72.

94. Law YM, Fielding JR. MRI of pelvic floor dysfunction: review. AJR Am J Roentgenol 2008;191(Suppl 6):S45–53.

95. Voderholzer WA, Schatke W, Muhldorfer BE, et al. Clinical response to dietary fiber treatment of chronic constipation. Am J Gastroenterol 1997;92(1):95–8.
96. Preston DM, Lennard-Jones JE. Severe chronic constipation of young women: 'idiopathic slow transit constipation'. Gut 1986;27(1):41–8.
97. Ramkumar D, Rao SS. Efficacy and safety of traditional medical therapies for chronic constipation: systematic review. Am J Gastroenterol 2005;100(4):936–71.
98. Wald A. Is chronic use of stimulant laxatives harmful to the colon? J Clin Gastroenterol 2003;36(5):386–9.
99. Muller-Lissner SA, Kamm MA, Scarpignato C, et al. Myths and misconceptions about chronic constipation. Am J Gastroenterol 2005;100(1):232–42.
100. Jones MP, Talley NJ, Nuyts G, et al. Lack of objective evidence of efficacy of laxatives in chronic constipation. Dig Dis Sci 2002;47(10):2222–30.
101. Xing JH, Soffer EE. Adverse effects of laxatives. Dis Colon Rectum 2001;44(8):1201–9.
102. Castle SC, Cantrell M, Israel DS, et al. Constipation prevention: empiric use of stool softeners questioned. Geriatrics 1991;46(11):84–6.
103. Chassagne P, Jego A, Gloc P, et al. Does treatment of constipation improve faecal incontinence in institutionalized elderly patients? Age Ageing 2000;29(2):159–64.
104. Johanson JF, Wald A, Tougas G, et al. Effect of tegaserod in chronic constipation: a randomized, double-blind, controlled trial. Clin Gastroenterol Hepatol 2004;2(9):796–805.
105. Kamm MA, Muller-Lissner S, Talley NJ, et al. Tegaserod for the treatment of chronic constipation: a randomized, double-blind, placebo-controlled multinational study. Am J Gastroenterol 2005;100(2):362–72.
106. Bouras EP, Camilleri M, Burton DD, et al. Prucalopride accelerates gastrointestinal and colonic transit in patients with constipation without a rectal evacuation disorder. Gastroenterology 2001;120(2):354–60.
107. Coremans G, Kerstens R, De Pauw M, et al. Prucalopride is effective in patients with severe chronic constipation in whom laxatives fail to provide adequate relief. Results of a double-blind, placebo-controlled clinical trial. Digestion 2003;67(1–2):82–9.
108. Camilleri M, Kerstens R, Rykx A, et al. A placebo-controlled trial of prucalopride for severe chronic constipation. N Engl J Med 2008;358(22):2344–54.
109. Johanson JF, Ueno R. Lubiprostone, a locally acting chloride channel activator, in adult patients with chronic constipation: a double-blind, placebo-controlled, dose-ranging study to evaluate efficacy and safety. Aliment Pharmacol Ther 2007;25(11):1351–61.
110. Heymen S, Jones KR, Scarlett Y, et al. Biofeedback treatment of constipation: a critical review. Dis Colon Rectum 2003;46(9):1208–17.
111. Chiarioni G, Whitehead WE, Pezza V, et al. Biofeedback is superior to laxatives for normal transit constipation due to pelvic floor dyssynergia. Gastroenterology 2006;130(3):657–64.
112. Rao SS, Seaton K, Miller M, et al. Randomized controlled trial of biofeedback, sham feedback, and standard therapy for dyssynergic defecation. Clin Gastroenterol Hepatol 2007;5(3):331–8.
113. Heymen S, Scarlett Y, Jones K, et al. Randomized, controlled trial shows biofeedback to be superior to alternative treatments for patients with pelvic floor dyssynergia-type constipation. Dis Colon Rectum 2007;50(4):428–41.
114. Harewood GC, Coulie B, Camilleri M, et al. Descending perineum syndrome: audit of clinical and laboratory features and outcome of pelvic floor retraining. Am J Gastroenterol 1999;94(1):126–30.

115. Nyam DC, Pemberton JH, Ilstrup DM, et al. Long-term results of surgery for chronic constipation. Dis Colon Rectum 1997;40(3):273–9.
116. Hassan I, Pemberton JH, Young-Fadok TM, et al. Ileorectal anastomosis for slow transit constipation: long-term functional and quality of life results. J Gastrointest Surg 2006;10(10):1330–6 [discussion: 36–7].
117. Gladman MA, Knowles CH. Surgical treatment of patients with constipation and fecal incontinence. Gastroenterol Clin North Am 2008;37(3):605–25, viii.
118. Knowles CH, Scott M, Lunniss PJ. Outcome of colectomy for slow transit constipation. Ann Surg 1999;230(5):627–38.
119. Rotholtz NA, Wexner SD. Surgical treatment of constipation and fecal incontinence. Gastroenterol Clin North Am 2001;30(1):131–66.
120. Kamm MA, Hawley PR, Lennard-Jones JE. Lateral division of the puborectalis muscle in the management of severe constipation. Br J Surg 1988;75(7):661–3.
121. Verne GN, Davis RH, Robinson ME, et al. Treatment of chronic constipation with colchicine: randomized, double-blind, placebo-controlled, crossover trial. Am J Gastroenterol 2003;98(5):1112–6.
122. Soffer EE, Metcalf A, Launspach J. Misoprostol is effective treatment for patients with severe chronic constipation. Dig Dis Sci 1994;39(5):929–33.
123. Roarty TP, Weber F, Soykan I, et al. Misoprostol in the treatment of chronic refractory constipation: results of a long-term open label trial. Aliment Pharmacol Ther 1997;11(6):1059–66.

Diarrhea and Malabsorption in the Elderly

Lawrence R. Schiller, MD[a,b,*]

KEYWORDS

• Diarrhea • Malabsorption • Aging effects on gut

SCOPE OF THE PROBLEM

Acute and chronic diarrheal disorders are common problems at all ages. It has been estimated that 5% to 7% of the population has an episode of acute diarrhea each year and that 3% to 5% have chronic diarrhea that lasts more than 4 weeks.[1] It is likely that the prevalence of diarrhea is similar in older individuals. The impact of diarrhea may be disproportionate in the elderly, many of whom are less fit physiologically to withstand the effect of diarrhea on fluid balance and nutritional balance.

Some of the impairment of physiologic fitness may be due to the effects of aging itself (eg, senescence of the immune system, age-related reduction in renal function, or nutritional status) and some is due to concomitant illnesses that cause or are complicated by diarrhea and that are more common in the elderly. For example, diabetes mellitus is more common as people grow older and diabetic neuropathy is more prevalent in diabetics with longer durations of disease. It is not unexpected that a complication of longstanding diabetic neuropathy, such as chronic diarrhea, might be seen frequently in older patients.

Keen observers have noted that some diarrheal diseases may present differently in the elderly than in younger patients. For example, celiac disease may present with extraintestinal symptoms such as cognitive decline or neuropathy that could be confused with other conditions.[2] It is essential that clinicians caring for older patients consider a broad differential diagnosis when investigating symptoms.

Diarrhea and malabsorption may have devastating effects on quality of life in the elderly. Fecal incontinence is a likely outcome when continence mechanisms that are "good enough" with formed stool are stressed by trying to hold back fluid stools (see the article by Leung and Rao in this issue). Malabsorption may tip the scales in elders with marginal nutritional status due to poor intake. Older patients are more likely

[a] Digestive Health Associates of Texas, 712 North Washington Avenue, #200, Dallas, TX 75246, USA
[b] Department of Internal Medicine, Baylor University Medical Center, 3500 Gaston Avenue, Dallas, TX 75246, USA
* Digestive Health Associates of Texas, 712 North Washington Avenue, #200, Dallas, TX 75246.
E-mail address: lrsmd@aol.com

Gastroenterol Clin N Am 38 (2009) 481–502
doi:10.1016/j.gtc.2009.06.008
0889-8553/09/$ – see front matter © 2009 Elsevier Inc. All rights reserved.

to be hospitalized with diarrhea, more likely to stay in the hospital longer, and more likely to die with diarrhea than younger patients.[3]

CHANGES IN INTESTINAL STRUCTURE AND FUNCTION WITH NORMAL AGING

Histologic studies of the intestinal mucosa published 30 years ago concluded that villous height and surface area declined in old age.[4,5] More recent investigation suggests that this is not the case and that there is no difference in jejunal mucosal biopsy specimens from old and young healthy subjects.[6] This is more in keeping with modern notions of epithelial biology in which epithelial cells are continuously replaced, turning over every 5 to 6 days.[7] As in the bone marrow, stem cells that produce enterocytes do not seem to wear out or become exhausted in the absence of disease over the course of a lifetime. Regardless of the age of the body housing the gut, the epithelium is eternally young.

This translates into maintenance of excellent epithelial function. In general, absorptive function is well preserved into old age. Absorption of D-xylose (when corrected for declines in renal function) is well maintained in a patient aged 80 years and declines only modestly thereafter.[8] The ability to absorb lactose in adult life (due to a gene-regulator mutation that is prevalent among individuals from the northern European gene pool) may decline with time but the mechanism for this is not clear.[9,10] There is no evidence that fat or protein absorption decreases with increasing age. Most micronutrients are absorbed well; the exceptions are calcium, folic acid, and vitamin B_{12}.

Calcium malabsorption may be more of a problem with inadequate vitamin D effect due to reduced sun exposure, vitamin D intake, or renal processing of vitamin D to active forms than an epithelial defect, although some evidence points to reduced epithelial sensitivity to vitamin D.[11] Folate malabsorption has been attributed to impaired luminal hydrolysis accentuated by achlorhydria or reduced folate conjugase activity.[12,13] Vitamin B_{12} levels tend to be lower in older subjects than in younger individuals, but this too may be multifactorial because direct measurement of radiolabeled cyanocobalamin absorption is normal.[14]

Salivary, gastric, biliary, and pancreatic secretory capacities are not diminished in healthy elders,[15,16] although there is some evidence that physiologic stimulation of secretion may be reduced. Changes in secretion may be related to changes in the regulatory systems of the gastrointestinal tract: the mucosal regulatory cell system, the enteric nervous system, or the immune system.

The mucosal regulatory system includes about a dozen types of enteroendocrine cells and so-called "brush cells" located in the epithelium.[17–20] These cells comprise about 10% of the epithelial cells in the gut and seem to be renewed along with the rest of the enterocytes from stem cells in the crypts. They have access to the lumen by the apical microvillar membrane and can sense physical and chemical characteristics of chyme within the lumen. In addition, these cells can respond to neurotransmitters released by nearby nerves.[19] The enteroendocrine cells respond by release of regulatory substances, such as serotonin and various peptides, into the subepithelial space and lumen. The brush cells respond by manufacture of nitric oxide which also has regulatory effects on nearby cells.[17] These regulatory substances can interact with local elements of the enteric nervous system, local effector cells by paracrine effects, and more distantly through hormone effects on other parts of the gut. Although some diseases have been associated with depletion of these cells,[21] there is no evidence that aging impairs their function.

The enteric nervous system is affected by aging, because like other neural networks, replacement of neurons is slow or nonexistent. Loss of neurons from the enteric nervous system begins in childhood and seems to accelerate as we grow older. It has been estimated that 40% to 60% of the enteric neurons are lost over a life-time.[22] The wonder may be that gastrointestinal function is as well preserved as it is. There may be greater loss of cholinergic neurons than nitrergic neurons, accounting for some of the motility changes that are observed as we age.[23]

Another regulatory system that may be affected by aging is the immune system. It is now known that immune cells release substances that affect gut function as well as modulate gut responses to infection.[24] Although evidence is scanty, the immune system may be less capable in the elderly, a concept known as "immunosenes-cence."[25] Immunosenescence may reflect an overall reduction in the ability to respond to infection with cellular and humoral effectors or a misdirection of the immune system against autoantigens, which may have something to do with the changes in the gut microbiota that have been observed with aging. Old people tended to have reduced populations of bifidobacteria and increased bacteroides.[26] The impact of these changes on susceptibility to enteric infection or on the occurrence of gastrointestinal symptoms has not been worked out. Potentially the bacterial flora of the gut might be manipulated to alter the mucosal immune response.[27]

ACUTE DIARRHEA IN THE ELDERLY
Infections

Acute diarrhea remains a common disorder in the general population with 6% of persons in 1 large sample having diarrhea in the 4 weeks preceding the survey (an annualized rate of 0.72 episodes per person-year).[28] Persons aged 65 years or older had a lower than average incidence (0.32 episodes per person-year). Older data suggest that the risk of hospitalization for gastroenteritis is twice as high for individuals aged 65 to 74 years and 4 times as high for individuals aged 75 years and older than in patients less than 50 years old.[29]

The usual bacterial, viral, and protozoal pathogens account for most of the identified cases of acute diarrhea.[3] These include *Salmonella*, *Shigella*, *Campylobacter*, *Clostridium difficile*, *Escherichia coli*, Norovirus, Rotavirus, *Giardia*, *Cryptosporidium*, and *Entameba histolytica*. In individuals with immunodeficiencies due to AIDS or immunosuppressive drug treatment (eg, corticosteroids, methotrexate, thiopurines, or antitumor necrosis factor biologicals) opportunistic infections with cytomegalovirus or herpesvirus should be considered. Older patients also travel more than in the past and so travelers' diarrhea may occur. In general, the presentations of these usual pathogens are similar to those seen in younger patients, and the course, treatment, and prognosis are similar to those of younger individuals.

Many older individuals reside in communal residences or nursing homes rather than in single family homes. This type of accommodation increases the opportunities for spread of infections if strict regimes to limit common source and person-to-person spread of infections are not in place. An excellent example of this phenomenon is pseudomembranous colitis due to *C difficile*.[30] Older individuals are more likely than younger adults to be hospitalized and to receive antibiotics for infections. They may become ill or be colonized with *C difficile* which they can bring into their residential institutions where it can spread widely in the environment.[31,32]

Older individuals are not only more likely to contract *C difficile* infection, but they are more likely to contract fulminant disease that may be fatal.[30,33] This may be due to impaired immune competence, comorbid illnesses, increased exposure to drugs that may predispose to infection (such as proton pump inhibitors), or to drugs that predispose to more toxic strains of *C difficile* (such as fluoroquinolones). Fulminant disease can be managed medically, but colectomy may be needed for unresponsive cases.[34]

Relapse of *C difficile* colitis also is more common in the elderly and seems to be increasing.[35,36] Risk factors for relapse include fecal incontinence, longer duration of fever, and treatment with H_2 receptor antagonists.[35] The proper management of relapsing disease is still undefined; in general, longer periods of antibiotic therapy are recommended, but novel therapies that replete the normal fecal flora or stimulate immunity are under development.[37]

Drugs

Because of the sheer number and variety of drugs consumed by people as they grow older, drug-induced diarrhea is a prominent cause of loose stools in the elderly.[38,39] If diarrhea begins soon after instituting a new drug, it is not too difficult to assign blame. To do this the physician must take a good drug history, not merely review a list of drugs that are being consumed. This history should include not only the drug and dose but also the timing of doses and any dose adjustments made over time.

Nearly half of the drugs listed in the pharmacopeia have diarrhea as one of their common side effects.[40] Common categories of drugs associated with diarrhea are presented in List 1.

List 1. Medications associated with diarrhea
   Acid-reducing agents (eg, histamine H_2 receptor antagonists, proton pump inhibitors)
   Antacids (eg, those that contain magnesium)
   Antiarrhythmics (eg, quinidine)
   Antibiotics (most)
   Anti-inflammatory agents (eg, nonsteroidal anti-inflammatory drugs [NSAIDs], gold salts, 5-aminosalicylates)
   Antihypertensives (eg, β-adrenergic receptor blocking drugs)
   Antineoplastic agents (many)
   Antiretroviral agents
   Colchicine
   Herbal products
   Heavy metals
   Prostaglandin (eg, misoprostol)
   Theophylline
   Vitamin and mineral supplements (eg, vitamin C, magnesium)

Tube Feedings

Another form of iatrogenic diarrhea that is common in the elderly is as a result of tube feeding.[41] This is most likely to occur with calorie-dense formulas infused directly into the small bowel and represents a variant of dumping syndrome. It may also occur with intragastric feeding, but this is less likely if normal regulatory mechanisms of duodenal control of gastric emptying are intact. Postulated mechanisms for tube feeding-associated diarrhea include hypertonicity-induced increases in intraluminal volume and motility, stimulation of gastrointestinal peptide release, and bacterial overgrowth. Slowing the rate of infusion, modifying the formula to increase fiber, or giving an antidiarrheal such as loperamide or diphenoxylate may mitigate the problem.[42]

CHRONIC DIARRHEA IN THE ELDERLY
Secretory Diarrhea

As in younger individuals, secretory diarrhea is the most common type of chronic diarrhea encountered.[1] Secretory diarrhea is almost always a result of reduced fluid and electrolyte absorption (rather than net secretion by the gut) related to inhibition of mucosal absorption rate or rapid motility that limits the contact time needed for complete absorption. The result of this is stools in which most of the osmolality is due to electrolytes (small osmotic gap, see later discussion).

There are many causes of chronic secretory diarrhea (List 2). Particularly in older patients, the thoughtful clinician first needs to consider systemic disorders that might be causing diarrhea before targeting primary gastrointestinal problems.

List 2. Differential diagnosis of secretory diarrhea in the elderly
    Ileal bile acid malabsorption
    Microscopic colitis
        Collagenous colitis
        Lymphocytic colitis
    Diverticulitis
    Drugs (see List 1)
    Disordered motility/regulation
        Diabetic autonomic neuropathy
        Irritable bowel syndrome (IBS)
        Postsympathectomy diarrhea
        Postvagotomy diarrhea
    Endocrinopathies
        Addison disease
        Carcinoid syndrome
        Gastrinoma
        Hyperthyroidism
        Mastocytosis
        Medullary carcinoma of the thyroid
        Pheochromocytoma
        Somatostatinoma
        VIPoma
    Idiopathic secretory diarrhea
        Epidemic secretory (Brainerd) diarrhea
        Sporadic idiopathic secretory diarrhea
    Laxative abuse (stimulant laxatives)
    Neoplasia
        Colon carcinoma
        Lymphoma
        Villous adenoma
    Vasculitis

Endocrine diseases

Diabetes is a prevalent problem for older patients. Diarrhea complicates the lives of about 20% of diabetics, making diabetes the most common systemic disease causing diarrhea.[43,44] The term, "diabetic diarrhea," should be restricted to diabetics with chronic secretory diarrhea. Steatorrhea can occur in diabetics, but is usually due to coexisting celiac disease, pancreatic exocrine insufficiency, or small bowel bacterial overgrowth. Diabetic diarrhea is considered to be a manifestation of autonomic neuropathy with decreased function of the adrenergic system and enteric nervous system.[45] Coexisting fecal incontinence can make diabetic diarrhea a nightmare for patients. Clonidine can be effective in diabetics with chronic secretory diarrhea, but opiate antidiarrheals work well also.

Addison disease is less common than diabetes among the elderly, but it is an important condition to consider in a differential diagnosis of chronic diarrhea because its systemic effects can be subtle.[46] The lassitude, fatigue, and weight loss characteristic of Addison disease may be ascribed to "old age" in the elderly, and electrolyte changes may be masked by concomitant use of diuretics for other medications. A cosyntropin stimulation test should be part of a second tier of investigations in patients with chronic diarrhea.

Hyperthyroidism also may not produce its full range of symptoms in the elderly. Patients may present with weight loss and diarrhea, but the adrenergic symptoms, such as tachycardia and tremor, may be absent. It is good practice to check the levels of thyroid hormone and thyroid stimulating hormone (TSH) in elderly patients with chronic diarrhea.

A group of endocrine problems that is rare at any age includes tumors secreting autocoids or gastrointestinal peptides. Although carcinoid tumors, gastrointestinal, and pancreatic endocrine neoplasms need to be considered in the differential diagnosis, they are so rare that measurement of plasma peptides and metabolites should only be done when the characteristic syndromes (eg, Zollinger-Ellison syndrome or carcinoid syndrome) are present, tumor is identified, or all other diagnostic tests have been negative.[47,48] Especially in the last situation, abnormal results are more likely to be false-positives rather than true-positives due to the rarity of these tumors.[49]

Drugs and iatrogenic diarrhea

As with acute diarrhea, drug therapy can cause chronic diarrhea.[39,40] Because older patients are treated with a bevy of drugs for therapeutic and preventative purposes, such complications can be common. Chronic diarrhea may result if drug interactions or declining renal function result in higher blood levels. Diarrhea may be due to a drug that the patient has taken for a while and the clear relationship between drug ingestion and initiation of diarrhea, as seen with acute drug-induced diarrhea, may be missing.

Older individuals are more likely than younger patients to have had surgeries or radiation therapy that may cause chronic diarrhea.[50,51] The therapeutic intervention may predate the onset of diarrhea by decades, but will have set the stage for chronic diarrhea. For example, gastrectomy may not cause diarrhea until the bacterial overgrowth that it encourages actually develops. Radiation enteritis likewise is a condition that may produce symptoms years after the treatment was completed.

IBS

IBS is the most common diagnosis made by clinicians in patients with chronic diarrhea, but it is an unlikely diagnosis for chronic diarrhea at any age, especially in diarrhea presenting for the first time in older patients. The salient symptom of IBS is abdominal pain; the diagnosis should not be made in patients without substantial abdominal pain or discomfort.[52] A category of "functional diarrhea" includes patients with painless diarrhea, but that diagnosis should be applied cautiously in the elderly, because most functional syndromes first present earlier in life and an alternate diagnosis can be made in most patients with continuous diarrhea. In the author's opinion functional diarrhea should be limited to those individuals with episodic or variable diarrhea in whom no alternative diagnosis can be reached.

Microscopic colitis

Lymphocytic colitis and collagenous colitis, the two varieties of microscopic colitis, are common in older patients.[53] In the general population, they are as common as Crohn disease, but the age distribution of microscopic colitis skews older, with a median age of onset of 68 years,[53] making it much more likely than Crohn disease as a cause of diarrhea in the elderly.

Although these diseases are inflammatory processes in the mucosa, the mucosa does not ulcerate, hence the typical findings of inflammatory diarrhea (blood and pus) are absent.[54] Microscopic colitis patients have the same HLA-D subtypes as celiac disease (DQ2, 8).[55] Presumably microscopic colitis is due to some luminal antigen, either dietary or microbial, that induces an increase in intraepithelial lymphocytes and in inflammatory cells in the lamina propria. The antigen is almost certainly not gluten. The only histologic difference between lymphocytic colitis and collagenous colitis is thickening of the subepithelial collagen band in the latter, the cause of which remains obscure.

The clinical history of microscopic colitis is characteristic: the gradual onset of watery, loose stools which can become moderately voluminous (typically 500–1000 g/24 h).[56] Stools are not bloody, pus and mucus are not typically present, and weight loss is gradual and minimal. In older individuals fecal incontinence is common, so much so that elderly patients with this presentation should have microscopic colitis at the top of their differential diagnoses.

The diagnosis of microscopic colitis depends on obtaining enough biopsies from the colon to allow the pathologist to make the diagnosis.[57] Most gastrointestinal pathologists are aware of the criteria for this diagnosis and so it should be missed rarely if biopsies are obtained. The trick is to remember to do this when the gross findings at colonoscopy are normal. One study suggested that this only happens about 80% of the time.[58]

Treatment of microscopic colitis is straightforward.[59] The best evidence is that budesonide is effective in collagenous colitis and probably lymphocytic colitis. Treatment should continue for 1 to 2 months at a dose of 9 mg daily. It can then be tapered off, but patients should be warned that the disease often relapses and further courses of treatment may be needed. Budesonide is not approved by the US Food and Drug Administration for this indication. Glucocorticoid side effects can occur in patients given budesonide, especially if they are receiving concomitant therapy with drugs that inhibit cytochrome P450 3A4. Weaker evidence supports the use of bismuth subsalicylate and cholestyramine in microscopic colitis.[60] Response rates with mesalamine or sulfasalazine are so low (~30%) that they should not be used for this indication. Diarrhea due to microscopic colitis usually can be controlled with opiate antidiarrheals and such therapy may be sufficient for some patients.

Bile acid diarrhea

It is well recognized that chronic diarrhea occurs when ileal dysfunction or resection results in delivery of a critically high concentration of bile acids into the colon (3–5 mmol/L).[61–63] Reaching this concentration depends on two offsetting trends: the extent of reduction of bile acid absorption by the ileum and not flooding the colon with fluid that tends to dilute bile acid concentrations. Patients with extensive ileal resections (>100 cm) deliver so much excess fluid to the colon that the critical concentration cannot be reached and diarrhea will not occur through a bile acid-mediated mechanism. Such patients may have diarrhea due to loss of surface area, but using bile acid-binding resins will not help.

Although this mechanism has been well worked out, the importance of bile acid malabsorption as a cause for chronic diarrhea is debated. In Europe, where a test for bile acid malabsorption (SeHCAT retention) is readily available, bile acid malabsorption is believed to be prevalent in chronic diarrhea and bile acid-binding resins are felt to be helpful in otherwise idiopathic diarrhea.[64] In the United States, research studies show that bile acid malabsorption is a common phenomenon in patients with chronic diarrhea, but therapeutic trials of cholestyramine have been unhelpful, with the results on stool weight not predicted by the extent of bile acid malabsorption.[65]

Nevertheless, bile acid-binders are of help in some patients with chronic secretory diarrhea and should be tried empirically when no diagnosis has been reached after study or when a bile acid-mediated diarrhea seems likely (eg, previous ileal resection or disease, previous cholecystectomy with predominantly morning diarrhea). The majority of the dose of bile acid-binder should be given at bedtime. Typically 4 g of colestipol, 4.5 g of cholestyramine, or 2.5 g of colesevelam should be tried initially at bedtime. Care must be taken to avoid coadministration with drugs that might be adsorbed by the resin.

Osmotic Diarrhea

Osmotic diarrhea is due to ingestion of some substance that is poorly absorbed and therefore results in retention of water within the lumen of the intestine.[66] The malabsorbed substances are either dietary components, such as disaccharides, or poorly absorbable ions, such as magnesium.

Lactose malabsorption is a true age-related condition. Lactose is the universal carbohydrate found in mammalian milk. Most babies are born with lactose phlorizin hydrolase (LPH, "lactase") in the brush border of small bowel enterocytes that has a high capacity to split lactose into its component monosaccharides, glucose, and galactose. These monosaccharides are then rapidly absorbed by the glucose-sodium cotransporter and are removed from the lumen. Some infants are born without active LPH and suffer with primary lactose intolerance. Like most mammals, most humans lose LPH activity after weaning, typically by the age of 20 years in humans. Some people maintain LPH activity into adult life as a result of a mutation in the gene regulator.[9,10] This results in the ability to digest and absorb lactose in adult life. This mutation is prevalent in the northern European gene pool and so the expectation in this population is that milk and dairy products can be consumed for a lifetime. Even in this population, however, the capacity for lactose hydrolysis declines with age and eventually may not be sufficient to hydrolyze all the lactose that is consumed. Those individuals then may develop symptoms, depending on the amount of lactose consumed.

Symptoms of lactose intolerance include excessive flatus and diarrhea.[10] The severity of these symptoms depends on the load of lactose consumed and the residual capacity for lactose hydrolysis. For every 10 g of carbohydrate that enters the colon, about 1 L of hydrogen gas and about 60 mmol of short chain fatty acids are produced by fermentation by enteric bacteria. Excessive flatus production can be seen with ingestion of relative small amounts of lactose in a lactose-intolerant person. Diarrhea depends on the absorbability of short chain fatty acids and their effects on colonic fluid absorption. The capacity of the colonic flora for fermentation of carbohydrate is about 80 g in the average adult and so unabsorbed lactose does not drive diarrhea directly until this threshold is exceeded.[67]

Older individuals may have always tolerated lactose and may not recognize that it is now causing their diarrhea. Clues to the diagnosis are the intermittency of symptoms (which depend on the amount of lactose ingested, which may vary from day-to-day) and the presence of flatus. Stool pH with carbohydrate malabsorption is acid (pH <6) and an osmotic gap may be present (typically >50 mOsm/kg).[66–68] Other carbohydrates, such as fructose, have limited capacity for absorption, and fiber is by definition not absorbable; concurrent ingestion of these substances may amplify symptoms in patients with lactose intolerance.

Other substances causing osmotic diarrhea are poorly absorbed ions, such as magnesium, sulfate, or phosphate. Magnesium is the prototype for this category. In addition to a small component of active absorption, 7% of the ingested load is absorbed passively, leaving 93% behind in the lumen to obligate water retention.[69] Thus stool output is directly proportional to load, accounting for magnesium's effectiveness as a laxative.

Patients with diarrhea may be taking poorly absorbed ions for therapeutic reasons or may ingest them inadvertently. For example, some calcium supplements or antacids contain magnesium and may induce diarrhea as a side effect. Other individuals may be taking laxatives to produce a factitious illness. Stools from patients with magnesium-induced diarrhea will have low concentrations of sodium and potassium, a high stool osmotic gap (>50 mOsm/kg), and high concentrations of magnesium.[69]

Inflammatory Diarrhea

Conditions that result in inflammation of the wall of the intestine and ulceration of the mucosa can cause blood and pus to appear in the stools, the fundamental characteristics of an inflammatory diarrhea (List 3). A brief differential diagnosis of this includes idiopathic inflammatory bowel disease, diverticular disease and diverticular colitis, ischemia, and neoplasia.

List 3. Causes of inflammatory diarrhea in the elderly
    Diverticulitis
    Infectious diseases
        Invasive bacterial infections (eg, tuberculosis, yersinosis)
        Invasive parasitic infections (eg, amebiasis, strongyloides)
        Pseudomembranous colitis
        Ulcerating viral infections (eg, cytomegalovirus, herpes simplex virus)
    Inflammatory bowel disease
        Crohn disease
        Ulcerative colitis
        Ulcerative jejunoileitis
    Ischemic colitis
    Neoplasia
        Colon cancer
        Lymphoma
    Radiation colitis

Idiopathic inflammatory bowel disease

Ulcerative colitis and Crohn disease are often believed to be diseases of young people. Although this is usually true, epidemiologic research shows that ulcerative colitis and Crohn disease occur with some frequency in older patients.[70,71] Although this was believed to be due to misdiagnosis, subsequent work has borne out this observation. The presentations and courses of inflammatory bowel diseases in the elderly are somewhat different than in younger individuals, but there is an overall similarity that makes them familiar.[72,73] A detailed review of this subject may be found elsewhere in this issue.

Diverticular disease and diverticular colitis

Diverticulosis is an age-related phenomenon that reaches epidemic proportions among the elderly. Up to 65% of people ≥65 years have diverticula.[74] This condition is asymptomatic in most patients. Five percent to 10% of people with diverticulosis may develop symptoms of diverticulitis or diverticular hemorrhage in their lifetime.[75]

Recently it has been recognized that some patients with diverticulosis develop a segmental colitis in the diverticula-bearing parts of their colons that may produce chronic pain and diarrhea.[76,77] The diagnosis depends on obtaining biopsies from the colon that show typical histopathologic findings. Treatment is undefined; most clinicians use mesalamine, but there is little direct evidence of benefit.

Ischemia

Ischemic colitis is an acute condition that produces bloody diarrhea and abdominal pain, usually in the left lower quadrant.[78] It seems to be due to low flow conditions in the inferior mesenteric artery and can be seen following circulatory compromise and as a side effect of certain drugs. It usually is self-limited, and in contrast to small intestinal ischemia, does not go on to produce necrosis and death. Diagnosis is made on the basis of sigmoidoscopy or colonoscopy.

Neoplasia

Colon cancer and lymphoma occasionally present with diarrhea.[79,80] Stools may have blood and pus in them due to mucosal ulceration proximal to an obstructing lesion. Large villous adenomas in the rectum may produce diarrhea due to excessive secretion of mucus from their surface.[81]

Fatty Diarrhea

The presence of steatorrhea implies problems with the solubilization of dietary fat by bile acids or malabsorption by the small intestine (List 4).[82,83] Isolated colonic pathology cannot produce steatorrhea. Certain conditions, such as small intestinal bacterial overgrowth, may be more common in the elderly.[84] Others that produce fatty diarrhea, such as celiac disease, may present atypically.[2,85]

List 4. Causes of fatty diarrhea in the elderly
    Malabsorption syndromes
        Mesenteric ischemia
        Mucosal diseases (eg, celiac disease, Whipple disease)
        Short bowel syndrome
        Small intestinal bacterial overgrowth
    Maldigestion
        Inadequate luminal bile acid concentration
        Pancreatic exocrine insufficiency

Celiac disease

The spectrum of celiac disease has expanded in recent years as criteria for the diagnosis have liberalized. Once considered only a disease of young people, celiac disease is now being diagnosed for the first time in some older adults.[85] The presentation of celiac disease may be more subtle, with accelerated osteopenia, hypoprothrombinemia, overshadowing diarrhea and weight loss.[2] A full treatment of this condition in the elderly can be found in the article by Rashtak and Murray in this issue.

Other mucosal diseases
Whipple disease, lymphangectasia, and other mucosal diseases do not seem to be especially prevalent in the elderly, but are sometimes diagnosed in older patients. With its wide variety of extraintestinal symptoms, Whipple disease can masquerade as decline in the elderly.

Pancreatic exocrine insufficiency
Malabsorption in older patients may be due to pancreatic exocrine insufficiency. In young adults it has been claimed that the pancreas secretes more than 10 times the necessary amount of enzymes to avoid steatorrhea. This margin may narrow in old age, but most cases of pancreatic exocrine insufficiency in the elderly seem to be due to chronic pancreatitis, although the cause of this may not be recognized. Alcohol-related pancreatitis is less common in the elderly than in younger adults. Late onset chronic pancreatitis produces less pain and progresses more rapidly to endocrine and exocrine pancreatic insufficiency.[86] Because pancreatic cancer may present with pancreatic exocrine insufficiency, patients with this diagnosis need a structural evaluation of the pancreas.[87]

Bile acid deficiency
Patients who do not deliver sufficient bile acid to the duodenum to solubilize fat develop steatorrhea due to incomplete fat digestion.[82] This can be seen with primary biliary cirrhosis or other causes of severe cholestasis and in patients with extensive ileal resections who cannot reabsorb bile acid. This cause of maldigestion is not always considered, but can be managed with bile acid supplements.[88]

Small intestinal bacterial overgrowth
Proper digestion and absorption in the small intestine depends on a germ-free environment. If bacterial counts build up, bile acid becomes deconjugated and can be absorbed from the lumen, lowering bile acid concentration and reducing fat absorption. Bacteria may disrupt the absorption of other nutrients, such as vitamin B_{12}, or may ferment carbohydrate substrates. Patients may develop abdominal bloating, pain, diarrhea, and weight loss.[89,90]

Bacteria can build up when stasis of luminal contents is due to structural problems such as jejunal diverticulosis or strictures, gastrocolic fistula, or upper tract surgeries. Small intestinal bacterial overgrowth (SIBO) also may develop with motility problems, such as seen with scleroderma, achlorhydria, or hypochlorhydria as seen with pernicious anemia or prolonged proton pump inhibitor therapy.

The frequency with which SIBO develops in older people is not clearly defined. Quantitative culture of luminal contents is deemed to be the gold standard test for SIBO with positive culture yielding greater than 10^5 bacteria/mL. Several different kinds of breath tests have been developed as "noninvasive" alternates, but technical issues mar performance statistics.[91] Abnormal tests seem to occur more frequently in the older population, but the clinical significance of this observation is not clear.

Patients with symptoms and positive tests for SIBO should be given a trial of antibiotic therapy.[90] A broad range of antibiotics has been used for this purpose, including trimethoprim/sulfamethoxazole, tetracycline, metronidazole, fluoroquinolones, and rifaximin. When steatorrhea is prominent, antibiotics that kill the anaerobic bacteria that deconjugate bile acids are recommended. Patients should receive a short course of therapy (10–14 days) and the impact of therapy on symptoms should then be assessed. If results are favorable, no therapy is needed until relapse occurs (as is likely because antibiotics do not treat the underlying problem predisposing to SIBO). If relapses are frequent, long-term suppressive therapy may be required. If there is no response to the initial course of therapy, an alternative antibiotic should be selected, based on sensitivity studies.

Mesenteric vascular insufficiency

Acute loss of blood flow to the small intestine is a life-threatening medical emergency. Chronic reduction of blood flow as seen with progressive atherosclerosis of the mesenteric arteries can produce a syndrome of pain and weight loss.[92] The pain is termed "intestinal angina" and occurs 1 to 3 hours postprandially. It is located in the periumbilical area and can be severe. Weight loss may be due to malabsorption, but is more likely due to sitophobia, avoidance of eating in an effort to limit pain. Diarrhea does occur sometimes. Diagnosis of this syndrome depends on recognizing the symptoms and their relation to meals in the setting of a patient with advanced atherosclerosis. Doppler sonography, magnetic resonance or CT angiography, or standard mesenteric angiography can be used for further evaluation. Revascularization or stenting can be used to treat this syndrome.

Diabetic steatorrhea

Diabetes can produce a watery diarrhea (see earlier discussion) or a fatty diarrhea.[93] Three causes should be sought if steatorrhea is identified in a diabetic: celiac disease, SIBO, and pancreatic exocrine insufficiency.

Post-surgical steatorrhea

Many different surgeries can predispose to the development of diarrhea or steatorrhea. Gastrectomy can result in dumping syndrome and often causes a 10% to 15% loss of body weight attributed to maldigestion.[50] Extensive small bowel resection will produce steatorrhea as a matter of course as the absorptive surface area is reduced.[94] The onset of diarrhea may be delayed as it may depend on development of aggravating factors, such as bacterial overgrowth.

Miscellaneous Diarrheas

Sometimes patients will report "diarrhea" when other processes are present that they cannot describe adequately. Identification of these processes is important because their management is different from the management of diarrhea.

Fecal impaction

Patients with constipation may develop a fecal impaction, a mass of stool that is too large to be passed through the anus.[95] Rectal distention causes relaxation of the internal anal sphincter and obstruction induces secretion proximal to the obstructing bolus. Liquid stool can flow around the impaction and may leak or be passed. The patient experiences loose stools that they report as diarrhea. A thoughtful digital rectal examination can identify impaction and should lead to effective treatment. Once the impaction is removed, the problem with loose stools should abate.

Fecal incontinence

Another condition that may be reported as "diarrhea" is fecal incontinence.[96] Many patients will not report accidental passage of stool without prompting and it is essential to ask patients about incontinence. Fecal incontinence is not due to voluminous diarrhea alone; there must be compromise of the sensory or muscle function that ordinarily preserves continence (see the article by Leung and Rao, elsewhere in this issue).

MANAGEMENT OF DIARRHEA AND MALABSORPTION IN THE ELDERLY
Diagnosis

The diagnostic approach to diarrhea in the elderly is fundamentally no different than in younger adults.[1] After taking a thorough history and performing a careful physical examination, the clinician should generate a differential diagnosis organized by likelihood of diagnosis.

The approach to acute diarrhea is fairly straightforward (**Fig. 1**). Infectious causes are most likely and can be investigated further, if needed, depending on epidemiologic considerations. Many experts suggest that bacterial cultures should only be done in patients with fecal leukocytes, because antibiotic treatment is limited to patients with invasive infections. Patients with any risk factors for *C difficile* infection should have an assay for toxin. Ova and parasite examination and fecal assays for protozoa (giardia and cryptosporidia) should be done selectively. The other causes for acute diarrhea can usually be distinguished by history.

In patients with chronic diarrhea, the differential diagnosis is much broader and so the direction of the diagnostic evaluation depends on the likelihood of the preliminary diagnosis.[97,98] In some situations, the likelihood of a specific diagnosis will be so high after reflecting on the history and physical findings that a specific diagnostic test can be done to prove the diagnosis and treatment can begin. In other situations, there is no overwhelmingly likely diagnosis and several competing diagnoses have roughly equal

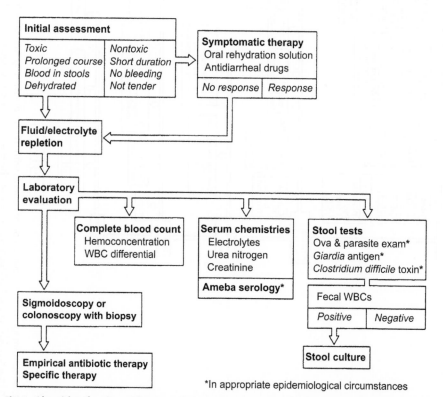

Fig. 1. Algorithm for the evaluation of patients with acute diarrhea. WBC, white blood cells. (*From* Schiller LR. Diarrhea. Med Clin North Am 2000;84:1259–74; with permission.)

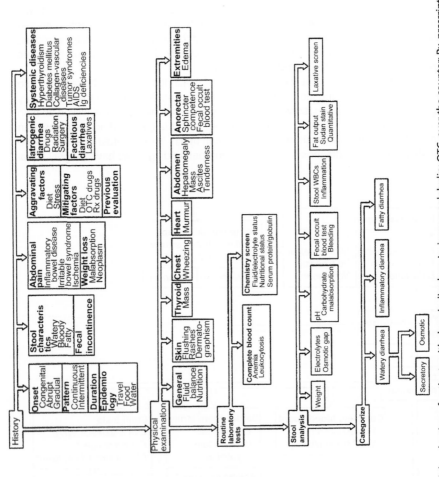

Fig. 2. Algorithm for the initial evaluation of patients with chronic diarrhea. Ig, immunoglobulin; OTC, over-the-counter; Rx, prescription; WBCs, white blood cells. (*From* Fine KD, Schiller LR. AGA technical review on the evaluation and management of chronic diarrhea. Gastroenterology 1999;116:1477; with permission.)

probabilities and thus a more extensive evaluation is required. In such circumstances it makes sense to categorize the diarrhea as being watery (secretory or osmotic), inflammatory, or fatty. This procedure simplifies the differential diagnosis and further evaluation can proceed more efficiently. An approach to the initial evaluation of a patient with chronic diarrhea is shown in **Fig. 2**.

If the diarrhea is watery, it is important to distinguish secretory from osmotic diarrhea. Osmotic diarrhea stops when the patient fasts and stops ingesting the poorly absorbed substance. Stool electrolyte analysis can be used to calculate the fecal osmotic gap.[68] In this calculation the sum of the sodium and potassium concentrations is doubled (to account for fecal anions) and subtracted from 290, the osmolality of colonic contents. If electrolyte concentrations are high as is the case with secretory diarrhea, the osmotic gap is small. If electrolyte concentrations are low as is the case with osmotic diarrhea, the osmotic gap is large and approximates the concentration of the poorly absorbed substance causing the diarrhea. The diagnostic evaluation can then proceed for either a secretory diarrhea (**Fig. 3**) or an osmotic diarrhea (**Fig. 4**).

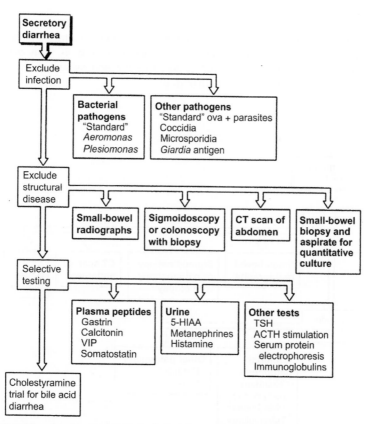

Fig. 3. Algorithm for the evaluation of chronic secretory diarrhea. ACTH, adrenocorticotropic hormone; 5-HIAA, 5-hydroxyindoleacetic acid; VIP, vasoactive intestinal peptide. (*From* Fine KD, Schiller LR. AGA technical review on the evaluation and management of chronic diarrhea. Gastroenterology 1999;116:1478; with permission.)

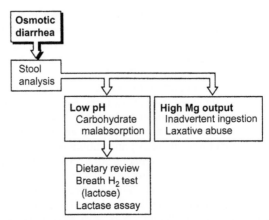

Fig. 4. Algorithm for the evaluation of chronic osmotic diarrhea. (*From* Fine KD, Schiller LR. AGA technical review on the evaluation and management of chronic diarrhea. Gastroenterology 1999;116:1478; with permission.)

If the diarrhea has characteristics of an inflammatory diarrhea, structural evaluation of the colon and small intestine should yield the diagnosis (**Fig. 5**). Fatty diarrhea is always due to small bowel or pancreatobiliary disease and evaluation focused on those organs is most likely to be helpful (**Fig. 6**).

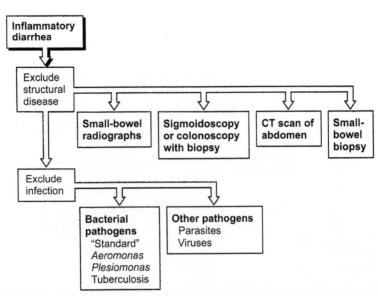

Fig. 5. Algorithm for the evaluation of chronic inflammatory diarrhea. (*From* Fine KD, Schiller LR. AGA technical review on the evaluation and management of chronic diarrhea. Gastroenterology 1999;116:1478; with permission.)

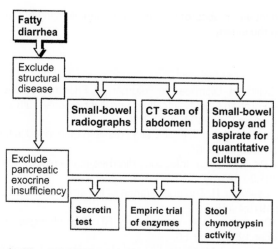

Fig. 6. Algorithm for the evaluation of chronic fatty diarrhea. (*From* Fine KD, Schiller LR. AGA technical review on the evaluation and management of chronic diarrhea. Gastroenterology 1999;116:1478; with permission.)

Treatment

Nonspecific treatment of older patients parallels that used in younger patients (**Table 1**), but certain nuances of treatment need to be observed.[99] Hydration is much more critical in the elderly. Because there may be pre-existing problems with renal or cardiac function, the rate of rehydration is critical: too fast and heart failure may be aggravated, too slow and azotemia may not be corrected. Potent narcotic antidiarrheals tend to be less well tolerated in the elderly; doses may need to be lower and should be adjusted more slowly. The potential for drug interactions is greater, making scrutiny of drug lists essential. Nutrition may be compromised rapidly by the

Table 1
Nonspecific therapy for diarrhea

Drug Class	Agent	Dose
Opiates	Codeine	15–60 mg qid
	Diphenoxylate	2.5–5 mg qid
	Loperamide	2–4 mg qid
	Morphine	2–20 mg qid
	Tincture of opium	2–20 drops qid
Adrenergic agonist	Clonidine	0.1–0.3 mg tid
Somatostatin analog	Octreotide	50–250 µg tid (subcutaneously)
Bile acid-binding resin	Cholestyramine	4 g daily to qid
	Colesevelam	1875 mg daily to bid
	Colestipol	4 g daily to qid
Fiber supplements	Calcium polycarbophil	5–10 g daily
	Psyllium	10–20 g daily

reduction in food intake or absorption that accompanies many of the conditions that cause diarrhea in the elderly.

REFERENCES

1. Schiller LR, Sellin JH. Diarrhea. In: Feldman M, Friedman L, Brandt LJ, editors. Sleisenger & Fordtran's gastrointestinal and liver disease. 8th edition. Philadelphia: WB Saunders Co.; 2006. p. 159–86.
2. Lurie Y, Landau DA, Pfeffer J, et al. Celiac disease diagnosed in the elderly. J Clin Gastroenterol 2008;42:59–61.
3. Slotwiner-Nie PK, Brandt LJ. Infectious diarrhea in the elderly. Gastroenterol Clin North Am 2001;30:625–35.
4. Webster SG, Leeming JT. The appearance of the small bowel mucosa in old age. Age Ageing 1975;4:168–74.
5. Warren PM, Pepperman MA, Montgomery RD. Age changes in small-intestinal mucosa. Lancet 1978;2:849–50.
6. Corazza GR, Frazzoni M, Gatto MR, et al. Ageing and small-bowel mucosa: a morphometric study. Gerontology 1986;32:60–5.
7. Ahuja V, Dieckgraefe BK, Anant S. Molecular biology of the small intestine. Curr Opin Gastroenterol 2006;22:90–4.
8. Webster SG, Leeming JT. Assessment of small bowel function in the elderly using a modified xylose tolerance test. Gut 1975;16:109–13.
9. Troelsen JT. Adult-type hypolactasia and regulation of lactase expression. Biochim Biophys Acta 2005;1723(1–3):19–32.
10. Lomer MC, Parkes GC, Sanderson JD. Review article: lactose intolerance in clinical practice—myths and realities. Aliment Pharmacol Ther 2008;27:93–103.
11. Armbrecht HJ, Zenser TV, Bruns ME, et al. Effect of age on intestinal calcium absorption and adaptation to dietary calcium. Am J Physiol 1979;236:E769–74.
12. Russell RM, Krasinski SD, Samloff IM, et al. Folic acid malabsorption in atrophic gastritis. Possible compensation by bacterial folate synthesis. Gastroenterology 1986;91:1476–82.
13. Baker H, Jaslow SP, Frank O. Severe impairment of dietary folate utilization in the elderly. J Am Geriatr Soc 1978;26:218–21.
14. Hyams DE. The absorption of vitamin B_{12} in the elderly. Gerontol Clin (Basel) 1964;55:193–206.
15. Gullo L, Priori P, Daniele C, et al. Exocrine pancreatic function in the elderly. Gerontology 1983;29:407–11.
16. Gullo L, Ventrucci M, Naldoni P, et al. Aging and exocrine pancreatic function. J Am Geriatr Soc 1986;34:790–2.
17. Lundgren O. Interface between the intestinal environment and the nervous system. Gut 2004;53(Suppl II):ii16–8.
18. Rindi G, Leiter AB, Kopin AS, et al. The "normal" endocrine cell of the gut: changing concepts and new evidences. Ann N Y Acad Sci 2004;1014:1–12.
19. Flemstrom G, Sjoblom M. Epithelial cells and their neighbors. II. New perspectives on efferent signaling between brain, neuroendocrine cells, and gut epithelial cells. Am J Physiol Gastrointest Liver Physiol 2005;289:G377–80.
20. Hansen MB, Witte AB. The role of serotonin in intestinal luminal sensing and secretion. Acta Physiol (Oxf) 2008;193:311–23.
21. Hogenauer C, Meyer RL, Netto GJ, et al. Malabsorption due to cholecystokinin deficiency in a patient with autoimmune polyglandular syndrome type I. N Engl J Med 2001;344:270–4.

22. Wade PR. Aging and neural control of the GI tract. I. Age-related changes in the enteric nervous system. Am J Physiol Gastrointest Liver Physiol 2002;283: G489–95.

23. Wade PR, Cowen T. Neurodegeneration: a key factor in the ageing gut. Neurogastroenterol Motil 2004;16(Suppl 1):19–23.

24. Kiba T. Relationships between the autonomic nervous system, humoral factors and immune functions in the intestine. Digestion 2006;74:215–27.

25. Sakamoto Y, Ueki S, Kasai T, et al. Effect of exercise, aging and functional capacity on acute secretory immunoglobin A response in elderly people over 75 years of age. Geriatr Gerontol Int 2009;9:81–8.

26. Hopkins MJ, Sharp R, Macfarlane GT. Variation in human intestinal microbiota with age. Dig Liver Dis 2002;34(Suppl 2):S12–8.

27. Guigoz Y, Dore J, Schiffrin EJ. The inflammatory status of old age can be nurtured from the intestinal environment. Curr Opin Clin Nutr Metab Care 2008;11:13–20.

28. Imhoff B, Morse D, Shiferaw B, et al. Burden of self-reported acute diarrheal illness in FoodNet surveillance areas, 1998–1999. Clin Infect Dis 2004;38(Suppl 3):S219–26.

29. Mounts AW, Holman RC, Clarke MJ, et al. Trends in hospitalizations associated with gastroenteritis among adults in the United States, 1979–1995. Epidemiol Infect 1999;123:1–8.

30. Zilberberg MD, Shorr AF, Kollef MH. Increase in adult *Clostridium difficile*-related hospitalizations and case-fatality rate, United States, 2000–2005. Emerg Infect Dis 2008;14:929–31.

31. Makris AT, Gelone S. *Clostridium difficile* in the long-term care setting. J Am Med Dir Assoc 2007;8:290–9.

32. McCoubrey J, Starr J, Martin H, et al. *Clostridium difficile* in a geriatric unit: a prospective epidemiological study employing a novel S-layer typing method. J Med Microbiol 2003;52:573–8.

33. McFarland LV. Update on the changing epidemiology of *Clostridium difficile*-associated disease. Nat Clin Pract Gastroenterol Hepatol 2008;5:40–8.

34. Jaber MR, Olafsson S, Fung WL, et al. Clinical review of the management of fulminant *Clostridium difficile* infection. Am J Gastroenterol 2008;103:3195–203.

35. Tal S, Gurevich A, Guller V, et al. Risk factors for recurrence of *Clostridium difficile*-associated diarrhea in the elderly. Scand J Infect Dis 2002;34:594–7.

36. Pepin J, Alary ME, Valiquette L, et al. Increasing risk of relapse after treatment of *Clostridium difficile* colitis in Quebec, Canada. Clin Infect Dis 2005;40: 1591–7.

37. Halsey J. Current and future treatment modalities for *Clostridium difficile*-associated disease. Am J Health Syst Pharm 2008;65:705–15.

38. Pilotto A, Franceschi M, Vitale D, et al. The prevalence of diarrhea and its association with drug use in elderly outpatients: a multicenter study. Am J Gastroenterol 2008;103:2816–23.

39. Ratnaike RN, Jones TE. Mechanisms of drug-induced diarrhea in the elderly. Drugs Aging 1998;13:245–53.

40. Abraham B, Sellin JH. Drug-induced diarrhea. Curr Gastroenterol Rep 2007;9: 365–72.

41. Luft VC, Beghetto MG, de Mello ED, et al. Role of enteral nutrition in the incidence of diarrhea among hospitalized adult patients. Nutrition 2008;24:528–35.

42. Shimoni Z, Averbuch Y, Shir E, et al. The addition of fiber and the use of continuous infusion decrease the incidence of diarrhea in elderly tube-fed patients in

medical wards of a general regional hospital: a controlled clinical trial. J Clin Gastroenterol 2007;41:901–5.

43. Shakil A, Church RJ, Rao SS. Gastrointestinal complications of diabetes. Am Fam Physician 2008;77:1697–702.

44. Quan C, Talley NJ, Jones MP, et al. Gain and loss of gastrointestinal symptoms in diabetes mellitus: associations with psychiatric disease, glycemic control, and autonomic neuropathy over 2 years of follow-up. Am J Gastroenterol 2008;103: 2023–30.

45. Chandrasekharan B, Srinivasan S. Diabetes and the enteric nervous system. Neurogastroenterol Motil 2007;19:951–60.

46. Tobin MV, Aldridge SA, Morris AI, et al. Gastrointestinal manifestations of Addison's disease. Am J Gastroenterol 1989;84:1302–5.

47. Modlin IM, Kidd M, Latich I, et al. Current status of gastrointestinal carcinoids. Gastroenterology 2005;128:1717–51.

48. Warner RR. Enteroendocrine tumors other than carcinoid: a review of clinically significant advances. Gastroenterology 2005;128:1668–84.

49. Schiller LR, Rivera LM, Santangelo WC, et al. Diagnostic value of fasting plasma peptide concentrations in patients with chronic diarrhea. Dig Dis Sci 1994;39: 2216–22.

50. Carvajal SH, Mulvihill SJ. Postgastrectomy syndromes: dumping and diarrhea. Gastroenterol Clin North Am 1994;23:261–79.

51. Davilla M, Bresalier RS. Gastrointestinal complications of oncologic therapy. Nat Clin Pract Gastroenterol Hepatol 2008;5:682–96.

52. Longstreth GF, Thompson WG, Chey WD, et al. Functional bowel disorders. Gastroenterology 2006;130:1480–91.

53. Pardi DS, Loftus EV Jr, Smyrk TC, et al. The epidemiology of microscopic colitis: a population based study in Olmsted County, Minnesota. Gut 2007;56:504–8.

54. Fernandez-Banares F, Salas A, Esteve M, et al. Collagenous and lymphocytic colitis. Evaluation of clinical and histological features, response to treatment, and long-term follow-up. Am J Gastroenterol 2003;98:340–7.

55. Fine KD, Do K, Schulte K, et al. High prevalence of celiac sprue-like HLA-DQ genes and enteropathy in patients with the microscopic colitis syndrome. Am J Gastroenterol 2000;95:1974–82.

56. Nyhlin N, Bohr J, Eriksson S, et al. Systematic review: microscopic colitis. Aliment Pharmacol Ther 2006;23:1525–34.

57. Lazenby AJ. Collagenous and lymphocytic colitis. Semin Diagn Pathol 2005;22: 295–300.

58. Harewood GC, Olson JS, Mattek NC, et al. Colonic biopsy practice for evaluation of diarrhea in patients with normal endoscopic findings: results from a national endoscopic database. Gastrointest Endosc 2005;61:371–5.

59. Chande N, MacDonald JK, McDonald JW. Interventions for treating microscopic colitis: a Cochrane Inflammatory Bowel Disease and Functional Bowel Disorders Review Group systematic review of randomized trials. Am J Gastroenterol 2009; 104:235–41.

60. Schiller LR. Pathophysiology and treatment of microscopic-colitis syndrome. Lancet 2000;355:1198–9.

61. Westergaard H. Bile acid malabsorption. Curr Treat Options Gastroenterol 2007; 10:28–33.

62. Robb BW, Matthews JB. Bile salt diarrhea. Curr Gastroenterol Rep 2005;7:379–83.

63. Hofmann AF, Hagey LR. Bile acids: chemistry, pathochemistry, biology, pathobiology, and therapeutics. Cell Mol Life Sci 2008;65:2461–83.

64. Wildt S, Norby Rasmussen S, Lysgard Madsen J, et al. Bile acid malabsorption in patients with chronic diarrhea: clinical value of SeHCAT test. Scand J Gastroenterol 2003;38:826–30.

65. Schiller LR, Bilhartz LE, Santa Ana CA, et al. Comparison of endogenous and radiolabeled bile acid excretion in patients with idiopathic chronic diarrhea. Gastroenterology 1990;98:1036–43.

66. Hammer HF, Santa Ana CA, Schiller LR, et al. Studies of osmotic diarrhea induced in normal subjects by ingestion of polyethylene glycol and lactulose. J Clin Invest 1989;84:1056–62.

67. Hammer HF, Fine KD, Santa Ana CA, et al. Carbohydrate malabsorption: its measurement and its contribution to diarrhea. J Clin Invest 1990;86:1936–44.

68. Eherer AJ, Fordtran JS. Fecal osmotic gap and pH in experimental diarrhea of various causes. Gastroenterology 1992;103:545–51.

69. Fine KD, Santa Ana CA, Fordtran JS. Diagnosis of magnesium-induced diarrhea. N Engl J Med 1991;324:1012–7.

70. Nguyen GC, Tuskey A, Dassopoulos T, et al. Rising hospitalization rates for inflammatory bowel disease in the United States between 1998 and 2004. Inflamm Bowel Dis 2007;13:1529–35.

71. Piront P, Louis E, Latour P, et al. Epidemiology of inflammatory bowel diseases in the elderly in the province of Liege. Gastroenterol Clin Biol 2002;26:157–61.

72. Wagtmans MJ, Verspaget HW, Lamers CB, et al. Crohn's disease in the elderly: a comparison with young adults. J Clin Gastroenterol 1998;27:129–33.

73. Greth J, Torok HP, Koenig A, et al. Comparison of inflammatory bowel disease at younger and older age. Eur J Med Res 2004;9:552–4.

74. Comparato G, Pilotto A, Franze A, et al. Diverticular disease in the elderly. Dig Dis 2007;25:151–9.

75. Stollman N, Raskin JB. Diverticular disease of the colon. Lancet 2004;363:631–9.

76. Freeman HJ. Segmental colitis associated with diverticulosis syndrome. World J Gastroenterol 2008;14:6442–3.

77. Lamps LW, Knapple WL. Diverticular disease-associated segmental colitis. Clin Gastroenterol Hepatol 2007;5:27–31.

78. Sreenarasimhaiah J. Diagnosis and management of ischemic colitis. Curr Gastroenterol Rep 2005;7:421–6.

79. Abella E, Gimenez T, Gimeno J, et al. Diarrheic syndrome as a clinical sign of intestinal infiltration in progressive B-cell chronic lymphocytic leukemia. Leuk Res 2009;33:159–61.

80. Gratama S, Smedts F, Whitehead R. Obstructive colitis: an analysis of 50 cases and a review of the literature. Pathology 1995;27:324–9.

81. Galanis IN, Dragoumis DM, Christopoulos PN, et al. Giant villous adenoma and McKittrick-Wheelock syndrome in an incarcerated rectal prolapsed. Colorectal Dis 2009, in press.

82. Schiller LR. Malabsorptive disorders. In: Grendel J, McQuaid K, Friedman S, editors. Current diagnosis and treatment in gastroenterology. 2nd edition. New York: McGraw-Hill Co.; 2002. p. 368–88.

83. Holt PR. Intestinal malabsorption in the elderly. Dig Dis 2007;25:144–50.

84. Riordan SM, McIver CJ, Wakefield D, et al. Small intestinal bacterial overgrowth in the symptomatic elderly. Am J Gastroenterol 1997;92:47–51.

85. Freeman HJ. Adult celiac disease in the elderly. World J Gastroenterol 2008;14:6911–4.

86. Gloor B, Ahmed Z, Uhl W, et al. Pancreatic disease in the elderly. Best Pract Res Clin Gastroenterol 2002;16:159–70.

87. Uomo G. Inflammatory pancreatic diseases in older patients: recognition and management. Drugs Aging 2003;20:59–70.
88. Gruy-Kapral C, Little KH, Fordtran JS, et al. Conjugated bile acid replacement therapy for short bowel syndrome. Gastroenterology 1999;116:15–21.
89. Meyers JS, Ehrenpreis ED, Craig RM. Small intestinal bacterial overgrowth syndrome. Curr Treat Options Gastroenterol 2001;4:7–14.
90. Ziegler TR, Cole CR. Small bowel bacterial overgrowth in adults: a potential contributor to intestinal failure. Curr Gastroenterol Rep 2007;9:463–7.
91. Schiller LR. Evaluation of small bowel bacterial overgrowth. Curr Gastroenterol Rep 2007;9:373–7.
92. Sreenarasimhaiah J. Chronic mesenteric ischemia. Best Pract Res Clin Gastroenterol 2005;19:283–95.
93. Ogbonnaya KI, Arem R. Diabetic diarrhea. Pathophysiology, diagnosis, and management. Arch Intern Med 1990;150:262–7.
94. Matarese LE, Steiger E. Dietary and medical management of short bowel syndrome in adult patients. J Clin Gastroenterol 2006;40(Suppl 2):S85–93.
95. Gallagher PF, O'Mahony D, Quigley EM. Management of chronic constipation in the elderly. Drugs Aging 2008;25:807–21.
96. Roach M, Christie JA. Fecal incontinence in the elderly. Geriatrics 2008;63:13–22.
97. Sellin JH. A practical approach to treating patients with chronic diarrhea. Rev Gastroenterol Disord 2007;7(Suppl 3):S19–26.
98. Schiller LR. Management of diarrhea in clinical practice: strategies for primary care physicians. Rev Gastroenterol Disord 2008;7(Suppl 3):S27–38.
99. Schiller LR. Review article: anti-diarrhoeal pharmacology and therapeutics. Aliment Pharmacol Ther 1995;9:87–106.

Fecal Incontinence in the Elderly

FelixW. Leung, MD, FACG[a], Satish S.C. Rao, MD, PhD, FRCP (LON)[b],*

KEYWORDS

- Fecal incontinence • Elderly • Nursing Home
- Community dwelling • Diagnosis and treatment

Fecal incontinence is a silent epidemic[1] among affected ambulatory patients; only about one-third of the affected individuals inform their care providers of the problem.[1] Factors associated with fecal incontinence include traumatic injury, neurologic deficits and inflammatory conditions of the anorectum, and defecatory disturbances associated with constipation and diarrhea.[2] Fecal incontinence is encountered in more than 50% of nursing home residents, and is associated with significant morbidity and use of health care resources.[3–5] A recent study of residents in skilled nursing facilities in Wisconsin[6] confirmed that dementia and advancing age were consistently associated with the development of fecal incontinence, but the strongest associations were impairment of activities of daily living and the use of patient restraints. In this review the authors discuss the problem of fecal incontinence in the community-dwelling elderly population and in nursing home residents.

FECAL INCONTINENCE IN COMMUNITY-DWELLING ELDERLY INDIVIDUALS

Fecal incontinence affects up to 20% of ambulatory community-dwelling elderly subjects.[1] Targeted treatment is based on addressing underlying pathophysiologic mechanism(s) as well as management focused on social or hygienic issues.[2]

Pathophysiology

Fecal incontinence is a consequence of many factors, and may result from deficits in internal or external anal sphincter or pelvic floor muscle function. The loss of endovascular cushions due to disruption of the hemorrhoidal plexus, impaired anorectal sensation associated with chronic constipation, poor rectal compliance and

Supported in part by VA Clinical Merit Research Funds (PI: Leung, Felix W.). Dr. Rao was also supported by NIH 2RO1-DK0570100-06A.

[a] Division of Gastroenterology, Department of Medicine, David Geffen School of Medicine at UCLA and Sepulveda Ambulatory Care Center, Veterans Affairs Greater Los Angeles Healthcare System, 111G, 16111 Plummer Street, North Hills, CA 91343, USA

[b] Department of Internal Medicine, University of Iowa Carver College of Medicine, University of Iowa Hospitals and Clinics, 200 Hawkins Drive, 4612 JCP, Iowa City, IA 52242-1009, USA

* Corresponding author.

E-mail address: satish-rao@uiowa.edu (S.S.C. Rao).

doi:10.1016/j.gtc.2009.06.007
0889-8553/09/$ – see front matter © 2009 Elsevier Inc. All rights reserved.

gastro.theclinics.com

compromised accommodation from aging, inflammatory bowel disease, radiation enteritis or pelvic surgery, or neuropathy affecting the pudendal, sacral, spinal, or central nervous system may contribute to fecal incontinence. In some patients incomplete evacuation of stool, large stool volume, liquid stool, and the irritant effect of bile salts in the rectum may also contribute to fecal incontinence.[2]

Management of Ambulatory Patients with Fecal Incontinence

An appraisal of a patient's history including potential predisposing factors, detailed drug history, particularly constipating drugs or excessive laxatives, and a systematic physical, neurologic, and rectal examination should provide vital clues that will facilitate management (**Fig. 1**). Therapy with a multilevel approach is outlined here.

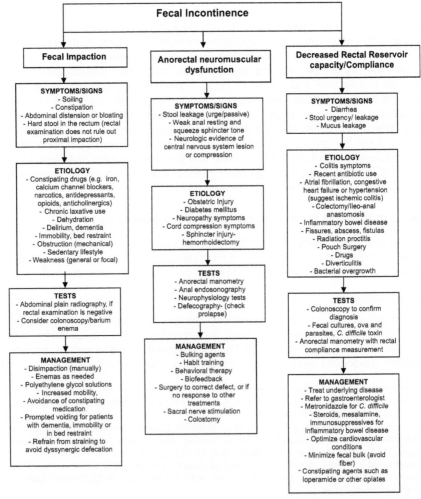

Fig. 1. Predisposing factors and algorithmic approach to the evaluation and management of fecal incontinence in an elderly subject.

Impacted stool requires manual disimpaction. If the stool is hard and difficult to expel, placing the patient on a regimen of controlled evacuation with suppositories or enemas at regular intervals may be necessary. Specific treatment of the underlying problem of diarrhea or constipation with increased fiber is important. Loperamide (Imodium) or diphenoxylate (Lomotil) dosed correctly will slow transit and solidify the stool.

Biofeedback has improved fecal incontinence in 50% to 67% of selected patients in controlled and uncontrolled reports and in short- and long-term studies. This behavioral approach consists of improving external anal sphincter muscle strength, rectal sensation, and rectoanal coordination.[7] A recent randomized, controlled trial of biofeedback as first-line treatment showed little advantage over conservative medical treatment,[8] but one long-term study showed significant improvement in patients who failed conservative treatment.[9]

Patients with fecal seepage have impaired rectal sensation and inappropriate elevation of anal sphincter pressure during defecation, particularly associated with "excessive" straining-induced inadvertent closure of the external anal sphincter.[10] Biofeedback to improve rectal sensation and timing of anal sphincter relaxation can ameliorate this symptom. A less labor-intensive approach of advising the patient to refrain from straining during defecation to avoid the development of obstruction to the outflow of the stool is logical, but has not been evaluated. Studies designed to establish efficacy and develop predictors of compliance with such a simple recommendation deserve to be assessed.

Fecal incontinence associated with rectal prolapse, rectovaginal fistula, or neurologic problems such as spinal cord injury may be amenable to surgery. The integrity of the anal sphincter and the intactness of rectal sensation can be determined by anorectal manometry. Anal ultrasound provides precise assessment of the integrity of external and internal anal sphincter muscles. Such objective anatomic data can facilitate more accurate reconstruction. Pudendal nerve terminal motor latency measures the neuromuscular integrity of the terminal portion of the pudendal nerve and the anal sphincter muscle. This test separates neuropathy (prolonged latency) from rectal wall disorders and provides an explanation for muscle weakness. Reconstructive surgery may not be successful in patients with pudendal neuropathy. Other surgical procedures include anterior repair, artificial bowel sphincter, and sacral nerve stimulation. Except for colostomy, none of these interventions (eg, external sphincter sphincteroplasty, pelvic floor muscle plication, neosphincter) can guarantee total continence. It is important that the patient is made aware of this limitation to minimize disappointment.[2]

Several reports were published in the past year describing efficacy of sacral nerve stimulation for treatment of fecal incontinence refractory to medical management.[11–16] One randomized, controlled study reported that sacral nerve stimulation was more effective than optimal medical therapy for severe fecal incontinence.[16] Patients (aged 39–86 years) with severe fecal incontinence were randomized to have sacral nerve stimulation (study group; n = 60) or best supportive therapy (control; n = 60), which consisted of pelvic floor exercises, bulking agent, and dietary manipulation. Full assessment included endoanal ultrasound, anorectal physiology, 2-week bowel diary, and fecal incontinence quality of life index. The follow-up duration was 12 months. The sacral nerve stimulation group was similar to the control group with regard to gender (F:M = 11:1 vs 14:1) and age (mean, 63.9 vs 63 years). The incidence of a defect of ≤120° of the external anal sphincter and pudendal neuropathy was similar between the groups. Trial screening improved incontinent episodes by more than 50% in 54 patients (90%). Full-stage sacral nerve stimulation was performed in

53 of these 54 "successful" patients. There were no septic complications. With sacral nerve stimulation, mean incontinent episodes per week decreased from 9.5 to 3.1 (P<.0001) and mean incontinent days per week from 3.3 to 1 (P<.0001). Perfect continence was accomplished in 25 patients (47.2%). In the sacral nerve stimulation group, there was a significant (P<.0001) improvement in fecal incontinence quality of life index in all 4 domains. By contrast, there was no significant improvement in fecal continence and the fecal incontinence quality of life scores in the control group. The investigators concluded that sacral neuromodulation significantly improved the outcome in patients with severe fecal incontinence compared with the control group undergoing optimal medical therapy. In one observational study, 4 (29%) of 14 patients (mean age 54 years, range 30–72) with disabling fecal incontinence resulting from obstetric injury did not have a significant benefit from temporary sacral nerve stimulation and 2 of these patients subsequently had a colostomy. The investigators concluded that sacral nerve stimulation offers improvement in continence and quality of life in patients with fecal incontinence whose other option might be a permanent colostomy.[13]

Management of the Social and Hygienic Aspects of Fecal Incontinence

Loss of self-esteem and self-confidence, disruption of relationships, and impairment of social and occupational activities are common in patients with fecal incontinence. Prompt changing of soiled pads or clothes, storage of soiled material in airtight containers, and appropriate hygienic measures can mask the odor associated with fecal incontinence. Perineal washes can disguise the smell of feces. Foods that can cause malodorous discharge vary from patient to patient, and limiting their consumption is prudent. For bedridden or unconscious patients with severe diarrhea, a fecal collection pouch, rectal tube, or anal plug device may be useful. Moist tissue paper (eg, baby wipes) that is not abrasive is preferable to dry toilet paper for cleansing of the perianal skin. Barrier creams (eg, menthol/zinc oxide ointment [Calmoseptine]) may prevent skin excoriations. Perianal fungal infection should be treated with topical antifungal agents (eg, clotrimazole [Mycelex]). When skin breakdown occurs, diversion of the fecal stream or changing the bedridden patient's position frequently is indicated. Scheduled toileting or prompted voiding with a commode at the bedside or a bedpan, and supportive measures to improve the general well-being and nutrition of the patient, may all play an effective supportive role.[2]

If incontinence is left untreated a host of dermatologic complications can occur, including incontinence dermatitis, dermatologic infections, intertrigo, vulvar folliculitis, and pruritus ani. The presence of chronic incontinence can produce a vicious cycle of skin damage and inflammation because of the loss of cutaneous integrity. Minimizing skin damage caused by incontinence is dependent on successful control of excess hydration, maintenance of proper pH, minimization of interaction between urine and feces, and prevention of secondary infection.[17] An anorectal dressing offers an effective, comfortable alternative to a pad for absorbing leaked feces that seems acceptable to men.[18]

FECAL INCONTINENCE IN NURSING HOME RESIDENTS

Fecal incontinence may be a marker of increased mortality and declining health in nursing home residents. In one study, 20% of nursing home residents developed new onset of fecal incontinence during a 10-month period after admission. Long-lasting incontinence was associated with reduced survival.[19]

Pathophysiology

Important risk factors associated with fecal incontinence in nursing home residents include immobility and dementia, which preclude residents from getting to the toilet in a timely fashion. Paradoxically the use of patient restraints was the most significant cause for the development of incontinence in nursing homes in one recent report, when the data were adjusted for the major reasons (dementia, blindness, arthritis, and stroke) to apply patient restraint and other risk factors for incontinence.[6] The development of fecal incontinence is one of the major risk factors for elderly persons who have been placed in the nursing home.[2] Impaction in the rectum with liquid stool leaking around the fecal mass is often associated with fecal incontinence in an elderly institutionalized person. When toileting assistance is not immediate, failure to perceive the arrival of stool in the rectum may produce severe urgency to defecate or leakage of stool.

Two studies that did not involve a toileting program have confirmed that dementia and immobility play a key role in the development of fecal incontinence. A retrospective study found that 46% of 388 nursing home residents were affected by fecal incontinence. Although diarrhea was the strongest risk factor, dementia actually played a greater role in the development of fecal incontinence.[3] Borrie and Davidson[20] also found that 46% of subjects (among 457 long-term care hospital patients) had fecal incontinence, and concluded that immobility and impaired mental function were independent predictors of fecal incontinence. Immobility was the strongest predictor of fecal incontinence as measured by nursing time spent toward assisting incontinent patients, and handling laundry and incontinence supplies.[20]

The role of these risk factors can be minimized by a prompted voiding program, even if residents have disorders that contribute to their fecal incontinence. Two studies have estimated the effectiveness of scheduled toileting programs in reducing the frequency of fecal incontinence. The results provided insight into the extent to which immobility and dementia contribute to this condition.[21,22] In one study, toileting assistance for urinary incontinence offered to male and female residents every 2 hours significantly decreased urinary incontinence and significantly increased the number of appropriate bowel movements from 23% to 60% (n=165).[22] Although the frequency of fecal incontinence was not decreased significantly, there was a trend in this direction. The second urinary incontinence treatment trial[21] involved a comprehensive intervention that integrated toileting assistance (prompted voiding), a fluid-prompting protocol, and exercises to improve mobility. Residents showed significantly decreased urinary incontinence, increased fluid intake, and improvement in mobility endurance. This program also resulted in a significant decrease in the frequency of fecal incontinence from 0.6 to 0.3 episodes per day and a significant increase in appropriate fecal voiding in the toilet. However, the frequency of fecal incontinence was only measured over 2 days and 46% of the residents had no fecal voids (continent or incontinent), revealing that constipation remained a persistent problem. The lack of a significant difference between the intervention and control groups in the total frequency of fecal voids during this 2-day monitoring period suggested that constipation was not alleviated by the intervention. Neither of these trials controlled for laxative use, medications with constipating side effects, or caloric intake that was known to be very low with consequent fiber intake that may have also been low. Also, anorectal function was not determined.

Several gastrointestinal disorders can play a role in the etiology of fecal incontinence in nursing home residents. Common causes are impaired anorectal sensation, lower sphincter squeeze pressures, and reduced integrity of sphincter or pelvic floor muscles.[23] One report described a subset of mentally intact but immobile nursing home residents—particularly stroke victims—who have fecal incontinence but have normal anorectal function. These residents require assisted toileting more than any other interventions. This small study compared anorectal measurements for four nursing home residents who had fecal incontinence, six ambulatory, elderly community-dwelling subjects who had fecal incontinence, and four controls without fecal incontinence.[23,24] Two of the four nursing home residents had normal measurements on anorectal testing, with normal squeeze duration and squeeze pressures. Despite having intact mental status and an awareness of impending bowel movement, both individuals had stroke-related impairment of their mobility and therefore required toileting assistance. However, the other two nursing home subjects had reduced squeeze pressures and other abnormalities compared with controls. The results suggest that although symptoms normally correlate with manometric abnormalities in ambulatory persons with fecal incontinence, such a correlation may not exist among immobile nursing home residents with fecal incontinence. An incorrect diagnosis of the factors influencing fecal incontinence may have a negative effect on the perception of nursing home residents regarding their management, and may partially account for the disparity between their observed symptoms and anorectal measurements.[23]

Constipation plays an integral role in the development of fecal impaction and fecal incontinence among the institutionalized elderly. The incidence of constipation increases with age and is also attributable to immobility, "weak straining ability," the use of constipating drugs, and neurologic disorders.[25] Defined as two or fewer bowel movements per week, hard stools, straining at defecation, or incomplete evacuation, constipation can result from a combination of lack of dietary fiber intake, poor fluid intake and dehydration, and the concurrent use of various "constipating" medications.[26] Fecal impaction, a leading cause of fecal incontinence in the institutionalized elderly,[27] results largely from the person's inability to sense and respond to the presence of stool in the rectum. Decreased mobility and lowered sensory perception are common causes.[28] A retrospective screening of 245 permanently hospitalized geriatric patients[29] revealed that fecal impaction (55%) and laxatives (20%) were the most common causes of diarrhea, and that immobility and fecal incontinence were strongly associated with fecal impaction and diarrhea.

Constipation, fecal impaction, and overflow fecal incontinence are common events in nursing home residents. Until recently, in the absence of comprehensive anorectal testing, drug-induced constipation was considered the likely explanation.[30] The high prevalence of constipation in nursing home residents, however, is only partly due to adverse drug effects.[31] Systematic anorectal testing of nursing home residents with fecal incontinence was reported in a recent study. This report documented impaired sphincter function (risk factor for fecal incontinence), decreased rectal sensation, and sphincter dyssynergia (risk factor for constipation and impaction) affecting up to 75% of the assessed residents.[32] The sphincter dyssynergia documented in these nursing home residents with fecal incontinence[32] sheds new light on the association between constipation and fecal incontinence in nursing home residents.

Treatment Options for Fecal Incontinence in Nursing Home Residents

When fecal incontinence is associated with diarrhea, it is important to treat underlying disorders. Conditions such as lactose malabsorption (or intolerance), bile salt malabsorption, and inflammatory bowel disease are treatable. Antidiarrheal medications, such as loperamide[33] and diphenoxylate,[33] or bile acid binders such as cholestyramine[34] may help. A gradual increase in the intake of dietary fiber can relieve constipation for many elderly patients. In a study of institutionalized elderly patients,[35] the use of a single osmotic agent with a rectal stimulant and weekly enemas to achieve complete rectal emptying reduced the frequency of fecal incontinence by 35% and the incidence of soiling by 42%. If fecal impaction is not relieved by laxatives and toileting, digital manual disimpaction may be necessary, followed by tap water enemas two or three times each week, and possible use of rectal suppositories.[36] The practice of routinely prescribing stool softeners, saline laxatives, stimulant laxatives, and single-agent osmotic products as prophylactic treatment against constipation and impaction deserves to be reexamined. In the presence of impaired sphincter function and decreased rectal sensation, the fluidity of the stool induced by the use of laxatives and stool softeners administered to prevent constipation and impaction may in fact predispose the nursing home residents to manifest fecal incontinence. The recent finding of anal sphincter dyssynergia in a high proportion of nursing home residents with fecal incontinence[32] suggests that a new approach to the management of fecal incontinence should consist of neuromuscular conditioning to improve the dyssynergic sphincter function. Even though the efficacy of biofeedback therapy has been demonstrated by a randomized, controlled trial in ambulatory patients,[37] in nursing home residents dementia and immobility may limit the effectiveness of such treatment. Hence, other novel approaches deserve to be considered. The approach using increased fibers[38] and prompted voiding[21] is a reasonable combination worth testing. Instructing the patients to refrain from straining to avoid dyssynergic defecation also seems logical. Nursing homes lack the staff and financial resources to provide residents with sufficiently frequent toileting assistance (including prompted voiding). These deficiencies need remedies.

Skin Care in Nursing Home Residents with Incontinence

The use of a skin care program that includes a cleanser and a moisture barrier is associated with a low rate of incontinence-associated dermatitis.[39] The use of a polymer skin barrier film three times weekly is effective in preventing incontinence-associated skin breakdown.[39] One uncontrolled trial described the use of an innovative adult brief that encouraged skin cleansing during incontinence care. The system was easily and effectively incorporated into the nursing home, and favored by certified nurse assistants whenever available (97% of the time). Patterns of incontinence care differed at follow-up, with the one-step incontinence system being compared with wipes placed at the bedside. This novel approach results in less linen used, fewer wipes used, and fewer interruptions of the certified nurse assistant during care.[40]

SUMMARY

Fecal incontinence in elderly patients is a challenging but treatable problem. In addition to local deficits such as weak sphincter muscles, impaired rectal sensation, and nerve damage, there are global issues such as impaired cognition, poor mobility, comorbid illness, and psychosocial effects. The associated embarrassment precludes many of the ambulatory patients from discussing the affliction with their care providers. The use of therapies that include an appropriate regimen of diet, fiber supplement, laxatives, enemas, drugs, scheduled toileting, biofeedback, sacral nerve stimulation, sphincter repair, and supportive care can minimize the severity and negative impact in ambulatory patients and nursing home residents with fecal incontinence.

REFERENCES

1. Johanson JF, Lafferty J. Epidemiology of fecal incontinence: the silent affliction. Am J Gastroenterol 1996;91:33–6.

2. Leung FW, Schnelle J, Rao SSC. Fecal incontinence. In: Capezuti EA, Siegler EL, Mezey MD, editors. The encyclopedia of elder care. New York: Springer Publishing Co.; 2008. p. 303–5.

3. Johanson JF, Irizarry F, Doughty A. Risk factors for fecal incontinence in a nursing home population. J Clin Gastroenterol 1997;24:156–60.

4. Harrington C, Carrillo H, Thollaug SC, et al. Nursing facilities, staffing, residents, and facility deficiencies, 1993 through 1999. San Francisco, CA: Department of Social and Behavioral Sciences, University of California; 2000.

5. Chiang L, Ouslander J, Schnelle JF, et al. Dually incontinent nursing home residents (clinical characteristics and treatment differences). J Am Geriatr Soc 2000;48:673–6.

6. Nelson RL, Furner SE. Risk factors for the development of fecal and urinary incontinence in Wisconsin nursing home residents. Maturitas 2005;52(1):26–31.

7. Rao SS, Welcher KD, Happel J. Can biofeedback therapy improve anorectal function in fecal incontinence? Am J Gastroenterol 1996;91:2360–6.

8. Norton C, Chelvanayagam S, Wilson-Barnett J, et al. Randomized controlled trial of biofeedback for fecal incontinence. Gastroenterology 2003;125(5):1320–9.

9. Ozturk R, Niazi S, Stessman M, et al. Long-term outcome and objective changes of anorectal function after biofeedback therapy for fecal incontinence. Aliment Pharmacol Ther 2004;20(6):667–74.

10. Rao SS, Ozturk R, Stessman M. Investigation of the pathophysiology of fecal seepage. Am J Gastroenterol 2004;99(11):2204–9.

11. Munoz-Duyos A, Navarro-Luna A, Brosa M, et al. Clinical and cost effectiveness of sacral nerve stimulation for fecal incontinence. Br J Surg 2008;95(8):1037–43.

12. Chan MK, Tjandra JJ. Sacral nerve stimulation for fecal incontinence: external anal sphincter defect vs. intact anal sphincter. Dis Colon Rectum 2008;51(7):1015–24.

13. O'Riordan JM, Healy CF, McLoughlin D, et al. Sacral nerve stimulation for fecal incontinence. Ir J Med Sci 2008;177(2):117–9.

14. Vitton V, Gigout J, Grimaud JC, et al. Sacral nerve stimulation can improve continence in patients with Crohn's disease with internal and external anal sphincter disruption. Dis Colon Rectum 2008;51(6):924–7.

15. Jarrett ME, Dudding TC, Nicholls RJ, et al. Sacral nerve stimulation for fecal incontinence related to obstetric anal sphincter damage. Dis Colon Rectum 2008;51(5):531–7.

16. Tjandra JJ, Chan MK, Yeh CH, et al. Sacral nerve stimulation is more effective than optimal medical therapy for severe fecal incontinence: a randomized, controlled study. Dis Colon Rectum 2008;51(5):494–502.

17. Farage MA, Miller KW, Berardesca E, et al. Incontinence in the aged: contact dermatitis and other cutaneous consequences. Contact Derm 2007;57(4):211–7.

18. Bliss DZ, Savik K. Use of an absorbent dressing specifically for fecal incontinence. J Wound Ostomy Continence Nurs 2008;35(2):221–8.

19. Chassagne P, Landrin I, Neveu C, et al. Fecal incontinence in the institutionalized elderly (incidence, risk factors, and prognosis). Am J Med 1999;106:185–90.

20. Borrie MJ, Davidson HA. Incontinence in institutions (costs and contributing factors). CMAJ 1992;147:322–8.

21. Schnelle JF, Kapur K, Alessi CA, et al. Does an exercise and incontinence intervention save health care costs in a nursing home population. J Am Geriatr Soc 2003;51:161–8.

22. Ouslander JG, Simmons S, Schnelle JF, et al. Effects of prompted voiding on fecal continence among nursing home residents. J Am Geriatr Soc 1996;44: 424–8.
23. Leung FW, Schnelle JF. Urinary and fecal incontinence in nursing home residents. Gastroenterol Clin North Am 2008;37(3):697–707.
24. Leung FW, Karyotakis NC, Rahman HU, et al. Fecal incontinence in a nursing home and an ambulatory population. Gastroenterology 1998;114:A778 [abstract].
25. Muller-Lissner S. General geriatrics and gastroenterology (constipation and fecal incontinence). Best Pract Res Clin Gastroenterol 2002;16:115–33.
26. De Lillo AR, Rose S. Functional bowel disorders in the geriatric patient (constipation, fecal impaction, and fecal incontinence). Am J Gastroenterol 2000;95:901–5.
27. Madoff RD, Williams JG, Caushaj PF. Fecal incontinence. N Engl J Med 1992;326: 1002–7.
28. Hirsh T, Lembo T. Diagnosis and management of fecal incontinence in elderly patients. Am Fam Physician 1996;54:1559–64.
29. Kinnunen O, Jauhonen P, Salokannel J, et al. Diarrhea and fecal impaction in elderly long-stay patients. Z Gerontol 1989;22:321–3.
30. Leung FW. Etiologic factors of chronic constipation: review of the scientific evidence. Dig Dis Sci 2007;52(2):313–6.
31. van Dijk KN, de Vries CS, van den Berg PB, et al. Constipation as an adverse effect of drug use in nursing home patients: an overestimated risk. Br J Clin Pharmacol 1998;46(3):255–61.
32. Leung FW, Beard MH, Grbic V, et al. Dyssynergia—key pathophysiologic mechanism for fecal incontinence (FI) in nursing home residents. Am J Gastroenterol 2007;102(S2):386 [abstract].
33. Harford WV, Krejs GJ, Santa Ana CA, et al. Acute effect of diphenoxylate with atropine(Lomotil) in patients with chronic diarrhea and fecal incontinence. Gastroenterology 1980;78(3):440–3.
34. Remes-Troche JM, Ozturk R, Philips C, et al. Cholestyramine—a useful adjunct for the treatment of patients with fecal incontinence. Int J Colorectal Dis 2008; 23(2):189–94 [Epub 2007 Oct 16].
35. Chassagne P, Jego A, Gloc P, et al. Does treatment of constipation improve faecal incontinence in institutionalized elderly patients? Age Ageing 2000;29: 159–64.
36. Whitehead WE, Wald A, Norton NJ. Treatment options for fecal incontinence. Dis Colon Rectum 2001;44(1):131–42.
37. Rao SS, Seaton K, Miller M, et al. Randomized controlled trial of biofeedback, sham feedback, and standard therapy for dyssynergic defecation. Clin Gastroenterol Hepatol 2007;5(3):331–8.
38. Khaja M, Thakur CS, Bharathan T, et al. "Fiber 7" supplement as an alternative to laxatives in a nursing home. Gerodontology 2005;22(2):106–8.
39. Bliss DZ, Zehrer C, Savik K, et al. An economic evaluation of four skin damage prevention regimens in nursing home residents with incontinence: economics of skin damage prevention. J Wound Ostomy Continence Nurs 2007;34(2): 143–52.
40. Al-Samarrai NR, Uman GC, Al-Samarrai T, et al. Introducing a new incontinence management system for nursing home residents. J Am Med Dir Assoc 2007;8(4): 253–61.

Diverticulosis and Acute Diverticulitis

John G. Touzios, MD, Eric J. Dozois, MD*

KEYWORDS

- Diverticulitis • Diverticulosis • Surgery • Management
- Complicated diverticulitis

Colonic diverticulosis is mainly an asymptomatic disease of Western countries, which first began to be recognized as a widespread problem in the 20th century. Infection and inflammation of these diverticula was first described in the late 1890s by Graser and later linked to the clinical symptoms in the early 1900s by Beer.[1,2] Most colonic diverticula are acquired, with the incidence increasing with age. Less than 2% of patients younger than 30 years old have diverticulosis, whereas more than 40% of patients older than 60, and 60% by age 80 years, acquire diverticula.[3,4] It is estimated that 10% to 25% of patients with diverticulosis go on to develop diverticulitis.[5] In the United States this results in approximately 130,000 hospitalizations per year and significant cost to the health care system.[6]

In 95% of cases, diverticula are located in the sigmoid and left colon. Right-sided colonic diverticula are rare in Western countries, although with increasing age there is a tendency for the diverticula to not only increase in number but also to develop more proximally in the colon.[7] In Asian countries, the main distribution of diverticula (up to 70%) is right-sided and may have a more genetic influence.[8]

The clinical picture for diverticulitis is one defined by a spectrum of presentations. Patients can present with a mild, isolated attack or can have severe and recurrent disease. In addition, a subset of patients present with complicated disease and some have "smoldering" disease. A new disease entity known as SCAD (Segmental Colitis Associated with Diverticula) has been described recently and may involve a different pathophysiology than classic diverticulitis.[9,10]

Not only has the etiology of diverticulitis become more complex than previously believed but the treatment algorithms have also evolved. The main components of treatment historically have been antibiotics and surgery. Less invasive nonsurgical procedures, along with new data suggesting the disease may not be as virulent as once believed, have recently questioned some of the surgical dogma that has guided treatment for many years.[11]

The authors have no disclosures.

Division of Colon and Rectal Surgery, Mayo Clinic, 200 First Street SW, Rochester, MN 66905, USA

* Corresponding author.

E-mail address: dozois.eric@mayo.edu (E.J. Dozois).

Gastroenterol Clin N Am 38 (2009) 513–525
doi:10.1016/j.gtc.2009.06.004
0889-8553/09/$ – see front matter © 2009 Elsevier Inc. All rights reserved.

gastro.theclinics.com

PATHOPHYSIOLOGY AND ETIOLOGY

Diverticula of the colon are not true diverticula (involving all three layers of the colonic wall) but pseudodiverticula, in which only herniation of the mucosal and submucosal layers is present.[12] Despite being commonly seen and treated, the exact etiology of diverticular disease remains unknown. The Industrial Revolution brought with it "roller milling," which removed up to two-thirds of the fiber content in foods, and the decrease in dietary fiber seen during this period correlates well with the beginning of symptomatic diverticular disease.[4] This led to wide support of the theory that lack of dietary fiber is the main cause of diverticulosis.[13–15]

A host of anatomic factors may work in conjunction with increased intraluminal pressures to lead to the pathogenesis of diverticula. Unlike other parts of the gastrointestinal tract, the colon is unique in that the outer muscular layer does not completely envelop it. The outer muscle layers coalesce to form 3 distinct bands, the taeniae coli, which run along the length of the colon. In addition, there are intrinsic weaknesses in the colon wall that develop where the vasa recta penetrate. The development of diverticula most commonly occurs along the mesenteric border of the antimesenteric taeniae, which corresponds to where the vasa recta are closest to the mesentery.[16–18]

Another structural difference in the colon of patients with diverticular disease relates to the thickness of the colon and the fact that collagen cross-linking increases with age.[19] This may in part explain why pan-diverticular disease develops in some patients (**Fig. 1**). It was initially believed that the colon became thickened with diverticular disease because of hypertrophy. On the contrary, follow-up studies revealed that microscopically there was no evidence of hypertrophy and that the changes were secondary to increased deposition of elastin.[20] This deposition results in highly contractile normal muscle, contributing to the increased luminal pressures. In addition, it has been shown that the amount of collagen cross-linking increases with age, especially in individuals older than 40 years.[19] As the cross-linking increases, the colon becomes more rigid, losing the compliance that is necessary to accommodate the increased pressures.

Segmentation is a phenomenon that occurs in the colon that leads to formation of isolated areas of extremely high intraluminal pressure.[18] Segmentation occurs when

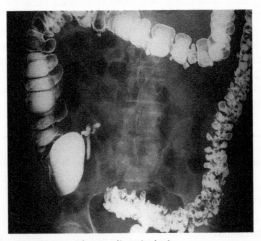

Fig. 1. Barium enema in patient with pan-diverticulosis.

two haustra that are near each other contract simultaneously and create a short segment of colon that is essentially a closed loop, leading to high pressures. This condition, along with studies demonstrating colonic hypermotility in the setting of diverticular disease, suggests that motility has some impact on the development of diverticula.[21,22]

The interplay of colonic wall structure, colonic motility, and the amount of dietary fiber likely leads to the formation of diverticula in the colon.[18] The etiology of why inflammation of the diverticula occurs and diverticulitis develops is not well understood. Symptoms from diverticulitis occur when there is microperforation or free perforation of a diverticulum. Following this event variable amounts of disease progression can occur, ranging from mild inflammatory changes to free perforation and abscess. The process that is poorly understood relates to the factors that lead to the perforation of the diverticulum. The predominant theory is based on inflammation being the main cause of perforation, although perforation can occur in the setting of no inflammation when high intraluminal pressures are present. There are many factors that most likely act in conjunction to cause the inflammation. Some of the factors implicated include obstruction of diverticulum, stasis, alteration in local bacterial microflora, and local ischemia.[18] Symptoms still may persist after there is documented resolution of inflammation. Heightened visceral hypersensitivity may account for some of the symptoms observed.[23] Studies have shown that colonic nerves may be damaged secondary to the inflammation, and this may lead to hyper-innervation and subsequently, persistence of symptoms.[24]

SYMPTOMS AND STAGING

Pain in the left lower quadrant associated with low-grade fevers, change in bowel movements, and mild leukocytosis are the classic clinical signs and symptoms of diverticulitis. A redundant sigmoid lying in the right iliac fossa occasionally can present with right-sided pain and thus be mistaken for acute appendicitis. Associated colonic symptoms can include obstipation, diarrhea, or increased mucus production. Abdominal distension secondary to ileus, as well as nausea or vomiting, can be present. Inflammatory processes that abut the bladder can lead to urinary urgency or frequency.

A pericolonic abscess secondary to perforated diverticulitis causes localized peritonitis. Involvement of the small intestine in a phlegmon can lead to obstruction. Fistulizing diverticulitis leads to specific symptoms related the organs involved. Colovesical fistulas can present as pneumaturia, fecaluria, or recurrent urinary tract infections. Enterocolonic fistulas have the potential to lead to severe diarrhea, especially if the small bowel involved is proximal. Passing stool through the vagina is the hallmark of colovaginal fistulas, and women with previous hysterectomy are at highest risk for fistula formation to the exposed vaginal cuff.

The vast majority of patients with diverticulosis are asymptomatic and therefore do not require any further treatment. Symptomatic patients can be subclassified into four main groups (Table 1). Complicated diverticulitis is defined as diverticular disease associated with obstruction, stricture, fistula, abscess, or perforation. Diverticular bleeding is usually not associated with diverticulitis and often presents as sudden and vigorous bright red lower gastrointestinal bleeding, which is usually self limiting. The Hinchey staging system has been used to differentiate severity of disease in the setting of acute diverticulitis associated with abscess (Box 1).[18]

Table 1 Clinical classification of acute diverticulitis	
Symptomatic Diverticulitis	Characteristics
Isolated, uncomplicated	Single episode of acute diverticulitis
Recurrent, uncomplicated (chronic)	Multiple, discrete episodes of acute diverticulitis
Complicated	Acute diverticulitis associated with abscess, fistula, obstruction, perforation, or stricture
Smoldering	Acute diverticulitis associated with ongoing, chronic symptoms

EVALUATION AND WORKUP

The workup of a patient suspected of having diverticulitis begins with thorough history taking and physical examination. It is important to try and characterize the pain and also assess for possible complications of the disease. Important history and symptoms to be elucidated include character and location of the pain, associated symptoms (fevers, chills, change in bowel habits, nausea, vomiting), and evidence of a complication (obstructive symptoms, pneumaturia, fecaluria, urinary tract infections, foul vaginal discharge). The differential diagnosis for lower abdominal pain that a practitioner should keep in mind includes appendicitis, urinary tract infection, irritable bowel syndrome, nephrolithiasis, gynecologic problems, infectious or ischemic colitis, inflammatory bowel disease, and malignancy.

Laboratory evaluation should include complete blood cell count with differential analysis and urinalysis.[25] The goal of imaging for acute diverticulitis is to define the location of disease, the extent of inflammation, and the presence of any complications. Multiple modalities have been used and studied in this setting, including plain radiographs, contrast enema, ultrasound, and computed tomography (CT). Barium enema is the most sensitive test to diagnose diverticulosis.[26,27] Although barium enema is an excellent test for defining luminal abnormalities of the colon, it does not visualize extraluminal manifestations of disease well.[28] Contrast studies may reveal extravasation of contrast, luminal narrowing, tethering, strictures, and fistulas.[29–31] In the presence of acute inflammation, only water-soluble contrast should be employed due to the risk of extravasation or perforation during the study. Barium peritonitis can be a life-threatening complication.

Box 1 Hinchey classification for diverticulitis
Stage I
Paracolic abscess confined to mesentery of colon
Stage II
Distant abscess in pelvis or retroperitoneum
Stage III
Purulent peritonitis
Stage IV
Feculent peritonitis

CT has become the imaging modality of choice for acute diverticulitis due to its sensitivity and specificity.[25,32–35] CT can assess intraluminal and extraluminal colonic pathology, evaluate the pericolonic tissue, define involvement of adjacent organs, and rule out other pathology such as appendicitis or gynecologic abnormalities (**Fig. 2**). Another aspect that makes CT the test of choice in assessing acute diverticulitis is that it allows for therapeutic intervention, such as percutaneous drainage of abscesses.

Cystography can be helpful to evaluate suspected colovesical fistulas, although these fistulas can be difficult to demonstrate radiographically.[25] Even if these fistulas cannot be visualized, the presence of acute diverticulitis and air in the bladder, in the absence of urinary instrumentation, is generally diagnostic for colovesical fistula. Endoscopy is another modality that is often considered in the workup of diverticulitis. However, most experts believe that colonoscopy or flexible sigmoidoscopy is not indicated in the acute setting, as there may be an increased chance of perforation or aggravating the inflammation.[36]

Following resolution of the acute diverticulitis episode it is vital to investigate the entire colon to rule out potential confounding diagnosis that can mimic diverticulitis, such as cancer or inflammatory bowel disease. About 3% to 5% of cases of diverticulitis are actually adenocarcinomas mimicking the symptoms of diverticular disease.[25,37,38] In addition to colonoscopy and barium enema, the use of CT colonography has increased in screening these patients for synchronous lesions.[39] CT colonography is equivalent to colonoscopy in identifying significant lesions in the setting of diverticular disease.[40] In addition, colonoscopy can be difficult in patients with extensive diverticular disease, and colonography would render colonoscopy unnecessary.

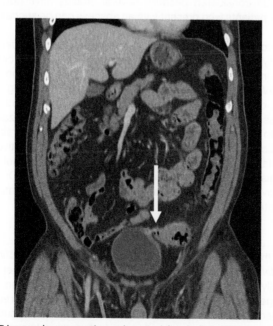

Fig. 2. Coronal CT image demonstrating colovesical fistula (*arrow*) in a patient with complicated diverticulitis.

MANAGEMENT OF DIVERTICULITIS
Medical Management

The mainstay of treatment of acute, uncomplicated diverticulitis is antibiotics, bowel rest, and analgesia. Antibiotics that cover gram-negative rods and anaerobic bacteria are typically prescribed for a 7- to 10-day period.[41] Oral antibiotics and outpatient treatment is appropriate when patients have mild symptoms, are capable of tolerating liquids, continue to have normal bowel function, and do not demonstrate evidence of complicated disease.[15,25]

Hospitalization may be required for severe cases of acute diverticulitis especially if the patient is unable to tolerate oral intake, has excessive vomiting, requires intravenous narcotics, or if symptoms and signs suggest escalating disease. Care must be taken in the elderly, as they may not tolerate outpatient treatment and may require closer observation for progression of disease.

Despite aggressive antibiotic therapy, some patients progress and require surgical intervention, and surgical consultation should occur early in the hospitalization. Recurrent episodes of diverticulitis, worsening symptoms despite medical treatment, the presence of complicated disease, and acute episodes in immunocompromised patients generally warrant surgical consultation.

Percutaneous Drainage of Diverticular Abscess

With the advent of image-guided percutaneous drainage, the management of perforated diverticulitis complicated by abscess has transitioned from an emergent surgical-based approach to a nonoperative, elective one. Pericolonic abscess accounts for up to 30% of cases of complicated disease.[11] Many investigators have shown that percutaneous drainage is successful in deferring the need for emergency surgical intervention.[42] If an interventional radiologist is available, this approach should strongly be considered because several studies have now demonstrated that up to 75% of patients who present with an abscess can be successfully managed this way.[43–45]

How long a percutaneous drain should remain in place is dependent on the size of the abscess cavity. Ideally, the drain is left in place until the cavity is collapsed and the fistula to the colon has closed. A weekly contrast study through the drain to assess collapse of the cavity may be required for large abscesses. The timing of surgical intervention following drain placement will depend on how quickly the local inflammatory response resolves. In addition to physical examination and normalization of leukocytosis, a follow-up CT scan is helpful 6 to 8 weeks following drainage to assure complete resolution of the inflammatory process. At this point elective surgical intervention can be planned. Colonoscopy to rule out other luminal pathology can also be safely done at this time as long as all inflammation has resolved. On rare occasions drains will not provide adequate local control of the sepsis and patients will still require urgent surgical intervention.

Elective Surgery

In recent years, the historical indications for elective surgical resection of recurrent, uncomplicated diverticulitis have been challenged.[11,25,46] The number of documented attacks historically was used as a benchmark for surgical intervention. Data published in the 1960s suggested that patients with multiple recurrent attacks responded less to antibiotics and had a higher risk of death from their disease.[3] More current data question the natural history of the disease as previously described. In a study by Chapman and colleagues,[11] most patients who presented with complicated diverticulitis had no antecedent attacks. Therefore, performing elective surgery after recovery from an uncomplicated episode of acute diverticulitis in an attempt to prevent a complication and decrease morbidity or mortality may not be justified.[37,47,48] The current American Society of Colon and Rectal Surgeons practice guidelines for the management of uncomplicated recurrent diverticulitis recommend that elective colon resection should be considered on a case-by-case basis.[25] The decision to proceed with surgery is based on several factors: the age of the patient, the comorbidities of the patient, the severity and frequency of the attacks, and the presence of ongoing symptoms after resolution of the acute attack. Some physicians currently use CT finding to "grade" the severity of disease and this may eventually prove to be the best indicator of the natural history of the disease following an attack.[32]

Unlike recurrent, uncomplicated diverticulitis, management of complicated diverticulitis is more straightforward. Colonic stricture, colovesical fistula, and pericolonic abscess may initially be managed conservatively, but ultimately surgical resection of the diseased sigmoid is recommended because long-term resolution of disease is unlikely. Some natural history studies on mesocolic versus pelvic abscesses have questioned whether small mesocolic abscesses need surgical intervention, as most respond to antibiotics and subsequent attacks may be less severe than once believed.[46]

With respect to age, it was previously believed that diverticulitis in the young is a much more aggressive disease and would inevitably lead to a higher risk of complications. Thus, past recommendations included offering surgery after one episode in patients younger than 50 years old.[49] This theory has been challenged by several current studies and it seems that diverticular disease in young patients acts in a similar way to that in the elderly.[47,50–52] There is, however, a higher cumulative risk of developing recurrent disease, as younger patients have a much longer life span than the elderly population. The current recommendation for the young should be as previously mentioned.[25]

Another subset that warrants special consideration for early surgical intervention is that of immunocompromised patients. For example, patients who are receiving chemotherapy, or are post transplant and on multiple immunosuppressive medications, are at increased risk of major complications from perforated diverticulitis. Moreover, emergency surgery in this cohort is associated with significant morbidity and mortality.[37] Therefore, elective resection should be considered in immunocompromised patients after a single episode.

The ultimate goal of elective surgery is to avoid the risks of recurrent diverticulitis and its associated morbidity and mortality. Recurrent diverticulitis can occur following surgery, and multiple variables have been studied to determine predictors of recurrence. The most significant predictor of recurrent disease following surgery is when the distal sigmoid (closest to the rectum) is not removed at initial resection. When the distal sigmoid is left in place and a colocolonic anastomosis is performed (versus a colorectal anastomosis), recurrent diverticulitis rates double. Benn and colleagues[53] showed, in 501 consecutive patients, that a colosigmoid anastomosis had a 12.5% incidence of recurrent diverticulitis versus 6.7% if the anastomosis was to the rectum.

Minimally Invasive Sigmoid Resection

Large abdominal incisions historically were required to perform sigmoid resection. With the emergence of new technology and innovative surgical perspectives, minimally invasive approaches to sigmoid resection have emerged and are now widely practiced.[54] Laparoscopic procedures use small abdominal wall trocars (5 mm) to access the abdomen so that vessel ligation, bowel transection, and anastomosis can all be performed entirely intracorporeally (**Fig. 3**). The only reason for abdominal wall incisions is to extract the colonic specimen, and new approaches can now use natural orifices such as the anus and vagina to extract specimens, negating the need for an abdominal wall incision and its associated morbidity.[55,56] Some surgeons are currently exploring the most advanced surgical technology available, the DaVinci robot, to perform sigmoid resection, and early results are promising.[57]

Using minimally invasive surgical techniques has resulted in significant patient-related benefits compared with the standard open approach. The short-term benefits of a minimally invasive approach are well established and include decreased pain, fewer pulmonary complications, decreased wound infection rate, less paralytic ileus, and shorter hospital stay.[58–60] Most reports are on patients with uncomplicated recurrent disease, although there has been increasing use of minimally invasive techniques in patients with complicated disease.[61,62]

Emergency Surgery

Less than 10% of patients require emergent sigmoid resection for complications of acute diverticulitis.[49] Emergency surgery is indicated for diffuse peritonitis, uncontrolled perforation, and failure of nonoperative management.[63]

The current standard surgical approach in an emergent setting is to remove the diseased colon, create a temporary end colostomy, and leave a closed rectal stump (Hartmann procedure). This procedure can then be followed by takedown of the colostomy and reanastomosis once the inflammation has resolved, usually 3 to 6 months after the initial surgery. However, the Hartmann procedure is not an ideal approach for multiple reasons: the takedown of the colostomy can be technically challenging, it involves a high morbidity rate, and a large proportion of patients, about one-third, will never have the colostomy taken down.[64,65]

Due to the high morbidity and mortality associated with the two-stage Hartmann procedure, many surgeons have transitioned to a one-stage approach whereby the sigmoid resection is done acutely along with a primary anastomosis. This approach

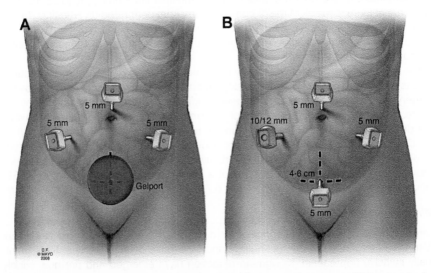

Fig. 3. Laparoscopic approaches. (*A*) Hand-assisted laparoscopic surgery. (*B*) Laparoscopic-assisted surgery. *Courtesy of* the Mayo Clinic, Rochester, MN; with permission.

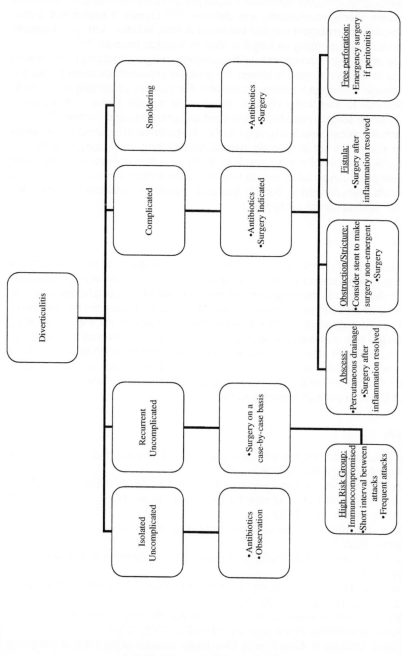

Fig. 4. Treatment algorithm for acute diverticulitis.

limits the number of operations needed and has been shown to decrease morbidity and mortality.[48]

However, the decision to proceed with primary anastomosis needs to be made on a case-by-case basis and involves many factors such as local tissue conditions, the comorbidities of the patient, and the operative stability of the patient.[15,38] Factors that are associated with poor outcomes include preoperative hypotension, acute renal failure, severe sepsis, malnutrition, and diabetes.[66,67] Overall, it seems that a one-stage approach for emergent surgical treatment is safe, feasible, and can potentially lower morbidity and mortality as long it is used in selected patients.[48,68]

Because of the high mortality rate with emergency surgery, bridging patients from emergency to elective surgery is always the goal. As previously described, percutaneous drainage is one such bridging approach. For patients presenting with colonic obstruction due to diverticular disease, endoluminal metallic stents to avoid emergency two-stage surgery have been described as achieving good success.[69]

Some small European studies have evaluated the potential of laparoscopic washout and drain placement for diverticular perforation requiring emergency surgery.[70–72] These studies have used this approach to avoid resection or Hartmann procedure in the acute phase, in an effort to make the resection a more elective procedure. To date the data seem promising, but this approach should be considered experimental until further studies can be performed.

SUMMARY

The management of diverticular disease will remain a challenge to physicians as the elderly population increases over the next decade. New and emerging technology will assist physicians in the diagnosis and management of the complications associated with acute and chronic diverticulitis. As more is learned about the natural history and pathophysiology of diverticular disease, treatment algorithms (**Fig. 4**) will likely evolve toward less invasive approaches. For patients that fail medical management, surgical management plays a critical role and can be associated with excellent results when done by experienced surgeons. Minimally invasive surgical approaches offer significant short-term benefits to patients and should be considered the standard approach for most patients requiring surgery.

REFERENCES

1. Beer E. Some pathological and clinical aspects of acquired (false) diverticula of the intestine. Am J Med Sci 1904;128:135–45.
2. Graser E. Das falsche darmdivertikel. Arch Klin Chir 1899;59:638 [German].
3. Parks TG. Natural history of diverticular disease of the colon. A review of 521 cases. Br Med J 1969;4:639.
4. Rafferty J. Diverticulitis. American Society of Colon and Rectal Surgeons core subjects; 2005.
5. Boles RS Jr, Jordan SM. The clinical significance of diverticulosis. Gastroenterology 1958;35:579.
6. Munson KD, Hensien MA, Jacob LN, et al. Diverticulitis. A comprehensive follow-up. Dis Colon Rectum 1996;39:318.
7. Hughes LE. Postmortem survey of diverticular disease of the colon. II. The muscular abnormality of the sigmoid colon. Gut 1969;10:344.
8. Nakada I, Ubukata H, Goto Y, et al. Diverticular disease of the colon at a regional general hospital in Japan. Dis Colon Rectum 1995;38:755.

9. Di Mario F, Aragona G, Leandro G, et al. Efficacy of mesalazine in the treatment of symptomatic diverticular disease. Dig Dis Sci 2005;50:581.
10. Tursi A, Brandimarte G, Giorgetti GM, et al. Mesalazine and/or *Lactobacillus casei* in preventing recurrence of symptomatic uncomplicated diverticular disease of the colon: a prospective, randomized, open-label study. J Clin Gastroenterol 2006;40:312.
11. Chapman J, Davies M, Wolff B, et al. Complicated diverticulitis: is it time to rethink the rules? Ann Surg 2005;242:576.
12. West AB, Losada M. The pathology of diverticulosis coli. J Clin Gastroenterol 2004;38:S11.
13. Burkitt DP, Walker AR, Painter NS. Dietary fiber and disease. JAMA 1974;229:1068.
14. Floch MH, White JA. Management of diverticular disease is changing. World J Gastroenterol 2006;12:3225.
15. Jacobs DO. Clinical practice. Diverticulitis. N Engl J Med 2007;357:2057.
16. Meyers MA, Volberg F, Katzen B, et al. The angioarchitecture of colonic diverticula. Significance in bleeding diverticulosis. Radiology 1973;108:249.
17. Slack WW. The anatomy, pathology, and some clinical features of divericulitis of the colon. Br J Surg 1962;50:185.
18. Thorson G. Benign colon: diverticular disease. In: Wolff F, Beck, Pemberton, editors. The ASCRS textbook of colon and rectal surgery. New York:Springer; 2007. p. 269.
19. Wess L, Eastwood MA, Wess TJ, et al. Cross linking of collagen is increased in colonic diverticulosis. Gut 1995;37:91.
20. Whiteway J, Morson BC. Elastosis in diverticular disease of the sigmoid colon. Gut 1985;26:258.
21. Bassotti G, Battaglia E, Spinozzi F, et al. Twenty-four hour recordings of colonic motility in patients with diverticular disease: evidence for abnormal motility and propulsive activity. Dis Colon Rectum 2001;44:1814.
22. Trotman IF, Misiewicz JJ. Sigmoid motility in diverticular disease and the irritable bowel syndrome. Gut 1988;29:218.
23. Simpson J, Scholefield JH, Spiller RC. Origin of symptoms in diverticular disease. Br J Surg 2003;90:899.
24. Stead RH. Nerve remodelling during intestinal inflammation. Ann N Y Acad Sci 1992;664:443.
25. Rafferty J, Shellito P, Hyman NH, et al. Practice parameters for sigmoid diverticulitis. Dis Colon Rectum 2006;49:939.
26. Gottesman L, Zevon SJ, Brabbee GW, et al. The use of water-soluble contrast enemas in the diagnosis of acute lower left quadrant peritonitis. Dis Colon Rectum 1984;27:84.
27. Hiltunen KM, Kolehmainen H, Vuorinen T, et al. Early water-soluble contrast enema in the diagnosis of acute colonic diverticulitis. Int J Colorectal Dis 1991; 6:190.
28. Fleischner FG, Ming SC. Revised concepts on diverticular disease of the colon. II. So-called diverticulitis: diverticular sigmoiditis and perisigmoiditis; diverticular abscess, fistula, and frank peritonitis. Radiology 1965;84:599.
29. Johnson CD, Baker ME, Rice RP, et al. Diagnosis of acute colonic diverticulitis: comparison of barium enema and CT. AJR Am J Roentgenol 1987;148:541.
30. Nicholas GG, Miller WT, Fitts WT, et al. Diagnosis of diverticulitis of the colon: role of the barium enema in defining pericolic inflammation. Ann Surg 1972;176:205.
31. Stein GN. Radiology of colonic diverticular disease. Postgrad Med 1976;60:95.

32. Ambrosetti P, Grossholz M, Becker C, et al. Computed tomography in acute left colonic diverticulitis. Br J Surg 1997;84:532.
33. Cho KC, Morehouse HT, Alterman DD, et al. Sigmoid diverticulitis: diagnostic role of CT—comparison with barium enema studies. Radiology 1990;176:111.
34. Gore RM, Goldberg HI. Computed tomographic evaluation of the gastrointestinal tract in diseases other than primary adenocarcinoma. Radiol Clin North Am 1982; 20:781.
35. Hulnick DH, Megibow AJ, Balthazar EJ, et al. Computed tomography in the evaluation of diverticulitis. Radiology 1984;152:491.
36. Chappuis CW, Cohn I Jr. Acute colonic diverticulitis. Surg Clin North Am 1988;68: 301.
37. Chapman JR, Dozois EJ, Wolff BG, et al. Diverticulitis: a progressive disease? Do multiple recurrences predict less favorable outcomes? Ann Surg 2006;243:876.
38. Dozois EJ. Operative treatment of recurrent or complicated diverticulitis. J Gastrointest Surg 2008;12:1321.
39. Hjern F, Jonas E, Holmstrom B, et al. CT colonography versus colonoscopy in the follow-up of patients after diverticulitis—a prospective, comparative study. Clin Radiol 2007;62:645.
40. Sanford MF, Pickhardt PJ. Diagnostic performance of primary 3-dimensional computed tomography colonography in the setting of colonic diverticular disease. Clin Gastroenterol Hepatol 2006;4:1039.
41. Ambrosetti P, Jenny A, Becker C, et al. Acute left colonic diverticulitis—compared performance of computed tomography and water-soluble contrast enema: prospective evaluation of 420 patients. Dis Colon Rectum 2000;43:1363.
42. Montgomery RS, Wilson SE. Intraabdominal abscesses: image-guided diagnosis and therapy. Clin Infect Dis 1996;23:28.
43. Ambrosetti P, Robert J, Witzig JA, et al. Prognostic factors from computed tomography in acute left colonic diverticulitis. Br J Surg 1992;79:117.
44. Neff CC, vanSonnenberg E, Casola G, et al. Diverticular abscesses: percutaneous drainage. Radiology 1987;163:15.
45. Stabile BE, Puccio E, vanSonnenberg E, et al. Preoperative percutaneous drainage of diverticular abscesses. Am J Surg 1990;159:99.
46. Ambrosetti P, Chautems R, Soravia C, et al. Long-term outcome of mesocolic and pelvic diverticular abscesses of the left colon: a prospective study of 73 cases. Dis Colon Rectum 2005;48:787.
47. Janes S, Meagher A, Frizelle FA. Elective surgery after acute diverticulitis. Br J Surg 2005;92:133.
48. Salem L, Veenstra DL, Sullivan SD, et al. The timing of elective colectomy in diverticulitis: a decision analysis. J Am Coll Surg 2004;199:904.
49. Stollman NH, Raskin JB. Diagnosis and management of diverticular disease of the colon in adults. Ad Hoc Practice Parameters Committee of the American College of Gastroenterology. Am J Gastroenterol 1999;94:3110.
50. Guzzo J, Hyman N. Diverticulitis in young patients: is resection after a single attack always warranted? Dis Colon Rectum 2004;47:1187.
51. Stollman N, Raskin JB. Diverticular disease of the colon. Lancet 2004;363:631.
52. Wong WD, Wexner SD, Lowry A, et al. Practice parameters for the treatment of sigmoid diverticulitis—supporting documentation. The Standards Task Force. The American Society of Colon and Rectal Surgeons. Dis Colon Rectum 2000; 43:290.
53. Benn PL, Wolff BG, Ilstrup DM. Level of anastomosis and recurrent colonic diverticulitis. Am J Surg 1986;151:269.

54. Vargas HD, Ramirez RT, Hoffman GC, et al. Defining the role of laparoscopic-assisted sigmoid colectomy for diverticulitis. Dis Colon Rectum 2000;43:1726.
55. Dozois EJ, Larson DW, Dowdy SC, et al. Transvaginal colonic extraction following combined hysterectomy and laparoscopic total colectomy: a natural orifice approach. Tech Coloproctol 2008;12:251.
56. Leroy J, Cahill RA, Asakuma M, et al. Single-access laparoscopic sigmoidectomy as definitive surgical management of prior diverticulitis in a human patient. Arch Surg 2009;144:173.
57. Weber PA, Merola S, Wasielewski A, et al. Telerobotic-assisted laparoscopic right and sigmoid colectomies for benign disease. Dis Colon Rectum 2002;45:1689.
58. Noel JK, Fahrbach K, Estok R, et al. Minimally invasive colorectal resection outcomes: short-term comparison with open procedures. J Am Coll Surg 2007; 204:291.
59. Schwenk W, Haase O, Neudecker J, et al. Short term benefits for laparoscopic colorectal resection. Cochrane Database Syst Rev 2005;3:CD003145.
60. Weeks JC, Nelson H, Gelber S, et al. Short-term quality-of-life outcomes following laparoscopic-assisted colectomy vs open colectomy for colon cancer: a randomized trial. JAMA 2002;287:321.
61. Jones OM, Stevenson AR, Clark D, et al. Laparoscopic resection for diverticular disease: follow-up of 500 consecutive patients. Ann Surg 2008;248:1092.
62. Schwandner O, Farke S, Fischer F, et al. Laparoscopic colectomy for recurrent and complicated diverticulitis: a prospective study of 396 patients. Langenbecks Arch Surg 2004;389:97.
63. Baxter N. Emergency management of diverticulitis. Clin Colon Rectal Surg 2004; 17:177.
64. Alanis A, Papanicolaou GK, Tadros RR, et al. Primary resection and anastomosis for treatment of acute diverticulitis. Dis Colon Rectum 1989;32:933.
65. Finlay IG, Carter DC. A comparison of emergency resection and staged management in perforated diverticular disease. Dis Colon Rectum 1987;30:929.
66. Krukowski ZH, Matheson NA. Emergency surgery for diverticular disease complicated by generalized and faecal peritonitis: a review. Br J Surg 1984;71:921.
67. Zorcolo L, Covotta L, Carlomagno N, et al. Safety of primary anastomosis in emergency colo-rectal surgery. Colorectal Dis 2003;5:262.
68. Constantinides VA, Tekkis PP, Athanasiou T, et al. Primary resection with anastomosis vs. Hartmann's procedure in nonelective surgery for acute colonic diverticulitis: a systematic review. Dis Colon Rectum 2006;49:966.
69. Small AJ, Young-Fadok TM, Baron TH. Expandable metal stent placement for benign colorectal obstruction: outcomes for 23 cases. Surg Endosc 2008;22:454.
70. Bretagnol F, Pautrat K, Mor C, et al. Emergency laparoscopic management of perforated sigmoid diverticulitis: a promising alternative to more radical procedures. J Am Coll Surg 2008;206:654.
71. Faranda C, Barrat C, Catheline JM, et al. Two-stage laparoscopic management of generalized peritonitis due to perforated sigmoid diverticula: eighteen cases. Surg Laparosc Endosc Percutan Tech 2000;10:135.
72. Franklin ME Jr, Portillo G, Trevino JM, et al. Long-term experience with the laparoscopic approach to perforated diverticulitis plus generalized peritonitis. World J Surg 2008;32:1507.

Intestinal Ischemia in the Elderly

John R. Cangemi, MD*, Michael F. Picco, MD, PhD

KEYWORDS

- Mesenteric ischemia • Elderly • Embolic
- Nonocclusive • Thrombotic

Ischemic disorders of the intestines are a rare disorder, accounting for less than 1 in every 1000 hospital admissions.[1] However, the mortality rate remains high, from 30% to 90%, largely related to delays in diagnosis in an elderly population with substantial comorbidities. Mesenteric ischemia occurs when blood flow to the intestinal tract on an acute or chronic basis is inadequate to support metabolic needs. It represents several different clinical presentations, including acute mesenteric ischemia (AMI), chronic mesenteric ischemia (CMI), nonocclusive mesenteric ischemia (NOMI), mesenteric venous thrombosis (MVT), and colonic ischemia (CI). Although varied in presentation, the end result is damage to the intestine, which may range from reversible ischemic changes to full thickness necrosis and death.[1–6]

PATHOPHYSIOLOGY

At rest the gut receives approximately 20% of the cardiac output. This amount increases to 35% after meal intake.[7] Three major vessels supply the intestines including the celiac axis, superior mesenteric artery, and the inferior mesenteric artery. Major branches of the celiac artery include the left gastric artery which supplies the stomach and duodenum. The remainder of the small bowel, right colon, and transverse colon are supplied by the superior mesenteric artery. The descending colon, sigmoid, and proximal rectum are supplied by the three branches of the inferior mesenteric artery. An extensive array of collaterals exist which protect the bowel from ischemic injury. These develop rapidly in response to a period of ischemia, and provide adequate perfusion for a variable period of time.[2] Collateral pathways include the gastroduodenal artery which represents an important potential connection between the celiac axis and the superior mesenteric artery. The marginal artery of Drummond and the arc of Riolan provide important collaterals between the superior mesenteric artery (SMA) and the inferior mesenteric artery. In addition to this, a network of intramural submucosal vessels exists which allows preservation of bowel

Division of Gastroenterology, Department of Medicine, Mayo Clinic Florida, 4500 San Pablo Road, Jacksonville, FL 32224, USA
* Corresponding author.
E-mail address: cangemi.john@mayo.edu (J.R. Cangemi).

Gastroenterol Clin N Am 38 (2009) 527–540
doi:10.1016/j.gtc.2009.06.002
0889-8553/09/$ – see front matter © 2009 Elsevier Inc. All rights reserved.

segments even in the face of reduced blood flow. However, there are areas which remain particularly vulnerable to an ischemic injury. The branches off the SMA form a series of arcades from which straight end arteries enter the intestinal wall limiting collateral flow. Also two "watershed" areas exist in the colon. These are Griffiths point, at the splenic flexure between the superior and inferior mesenteric arteries, and Sudeck point in the rectosigmoid between the inferior mesenteric and the hypogastric arteries. These areas are vulnerable secondary to incomplete anastomoses of the marginal artery in these areas.

This article reviews the clinical spectrum of mesenteric ischemia in the elderly with particular emphasis on the varied presentations, evaluation, and management of ischemic disorders of the intestines.

ACUTE MESENTERIC ISCHEMIA

AMI remains a potentially lethal disorder with little improvement in survival in the past 70 years. Average mortality approaches 71% with a range of 59% to 93%.[2] The lack of progress relates to the delay in diagnosis with only one third of patients properly diagnosed before surgical intervention or death.[8] This suggests that mortality may even be higher as many fatal cases may go unrecognized.[9] It is essential then to maintain a high index of suspicion in an elderly patient who presents with acute abdominal pain and has associated risk factors for vascular disease. Classically the pain at presentation is out of proportion to the physical findings.[1–3,10] In fact any development of peritoneal signs suggests the onset of transmural infarction which portends a dismal prognosis. Other presenting complaints include nausea and vomiting, abdominal distention, or forceful diarrhea which may be dark or test positive for blood. However, in the elderly the presentation may differ somewhat with less frequent abdominal pain and more often symptoms such as tachypnea or mental status changes. These are nonspecific symptoms, but when coupled with the clinical history, should alert the clinician to the diagnosis. Patients at particular risk for AMI include those over the age of 60 with a history of cardiomyopathy, cardiac arrhythmias, myocardial infarction, renal failure (hemodialysis), hypotension, hypovolemia, ventricular aneurysms, hypercoagulable state, or use of vasoactive drugs.

The mortality rate is entirely dependent on early diagnosis. In one series, survival decreased from 100% to 18% if the diagnosis were delayed from less than 12 hours to greater than 24 hours.[11] Distinguishing this condition from a differential diagnosis which includes inflammatory bowel disease, diverticulitis, small bowel obstruction, acute pancreatitis, peptic ulcer disease, appendicitis, cholecystitis, or infectious gastroenteritis may be difficult as these conditions are far more common than mesenteric ischemia.[12] Early on, the laboratory assessment is of little value in distinguishing among these diagnoses. Common findings include leukocytosis, hemoconcentration, elevated amylase levels, abnormal liver enzymes (aspartate aminotransferase [AST], alkaline phosphatase), hyperphosphatemia, and metabolic acidosis. Unfortunately none of these findings is specific for ischemia and more characteristic abnormalities such as elevated lactic acid levels appear later in the course, after the onset of infarction. D-Dimer may have value in detecting early ischemia, but remains to be confirmed.[13]

A plain film of the abdomen is typically normal early on, with less than 40% of patients demonstrating the characteristic findings of "thumbprinting" or thickening of bowel loops. As with the laboratory results, changes on the flat plate occur later, indicating a poorer outcome. In one study, a normal flat plate was associated with a mortality of 29%, compared with 78% if pathologic changes were seen.[14]

Arterial Embolism

Arterial embolism is the most common cause for ischemia accounting for 40% to 50% of cases of AMI. It also carries a poor prognosis with a mortality rate of approximately 70%. The onset of symptoms is rapid, as the acute occlusion allows little time for development of collaterals. Emboli have a specific predilection for the SMA because it emerges from the aorta at an oblique angle. The emboli typically lodge distal to the origin of the middle colic artery which then spares the duodenum and proximal jejunum. This characteristic helps to distinguish it from arterial thrombosis which often has a more proximal extent. Most emboli arise from a cardiac source including atrial fibrillation, myocardial infarct (MI), and structural heart defects such as a right-to-left shunt or a ventricular aneurysm. In a review of autopsy findings in 122 patients with embolus to the SMA 86 patients (70%) were documented to have a cardiac source.[15] In 83 of these patients (68%) synchronous emboli were found, emphasizing the long-term risk the survivors face. In nearly one third of patients who present with arterial emboli, there is a history of a previous embolic event.

Arterial Thrombosis

Arterial thrombosis accounts for 25% to 30% of episodes of AMI and may carry the worst prognosis with mortality approaching 90%.[1,5] This high mortality relates to the extent of bowel necrosis as, most often, thrombosis involves the origin of the SMA. Most patients with this diagnosis have advanced atherosclerotic disease and will give an antecedent history of CMI. The onset is more insidious as there is adequate time to develop an array of collateral vessels. Ischemia occurs with the occlusion of a major vessel or collateral.

MESENTERIC VENOUS THROMBOSIS

MVT is the least common cause of mesenteric ischemia, accounting for approximately 10% of cases. However, mortality remains high at between 20% and 50%. Most cases have an identifiable cause with only 10% now characterized as idiopathic. These causes include cirrhosis with portal hypertension, a hypercoagulable state due to inherent clotting disorders including factor V Leiden mutation, protein C or protein S deficiency, malignancy, or recent surgery. Up to 50% of cases have had a deep venous thrombosis or pulmonary embolism before.[16] Bowel involvement in MVT is usually segmental with edema and hemorrhage of the bowel wall with focal exfoliation of the mucosa. Its presentation may be acute or chronic, generally presenting for evaluation 1 to 2 weeks after onset of symptoms. The diagnosis is difficult as the symptoms are often nonspecific. Most patients will have abdominal pain (90%), but the onset is variable and location is inconsistent. Patients typically do not experience the classic symptoms of postprandial pain and sitophobia seen in arterial thrombosis. Nausea and vomiting are present in 60% to 75% of patients and 30% will have altered bowel habits with either constipation or diarrhea. The diarrhea infrequently is bloody, but more than one half of patients are positive for occult blood. Fever is a common finding along with abdominal tenderness, distention with decreased bowel sounds, but peritoneal signs are seen in only two thirds of patients.

As with AMI, the laboratory parameters are nonspecific. Plain films of the abdomen often are normal at presentation or simply show a nonspecific ileus. These factors all contribute to the difficulty in making this diagnosis, but do not lessen the importance. Mortality is directly related to timing of diagnosis and institution of prompt therapy, as discussed in this article.

NONOCCLUSIVE MESENTERIC ISCHEMIA

NOMI accounts for 20% to 30% of acute mesenteric ischemic events, and, as with other types of AMI, carries a high mortality rate of 50% to 90%. NOMI refers to ischemia secondary to a low flow state in the absence of arterial or venous occlusion. The decrease in cardiac output is associated with a diffuse mesenteric vasoconstriction which further reduces flow, leading to ischemia and ultimately necrosis. Clinical symptoms are often missed as the patients with NOMI may be critically ill and the onset of symptoms is often insidious. Any condition associated with reduced cardiac output may cause NOMI, for example, MI, congestive heart failure, hypovolemia, or hypotension. Use of alpha-adrenergic agonists, digoxin or beta-receptor blocking agents may also increase risk. NOMI is also seen in the setting of major abdominal or cardiovascular surgery. The risk increases further if the patients are receiving enteral nutrition. The increased demand generated by the enteral feedings may exceed the capacity of blood flow to meet the metabolic requirements. Incidence of NOMI in this setting has been reported to be 0.3% to 8.5%.[17]

A series of autopsies were reviewed to assess the incidence of NOMI, the extent of involvement, and the potential risk factors.[18] The incidence was rare, yet increased in octogenarians from 2/100,000 person-years before age 80 to 40/100,000 person-years after age 80. Only 29% were correctly diagnosed before death, again verifying the difficulty in making an early diagnosis. The 3 major potential causes in this series were heart failure, atrial fibrillation, and recent major surgery. Forty percent of fatal cases of NOMI were found to have mesenteric stenosis which further contributed to the low flow state.

As with other forms of AMI, early laboratories and the abdominal flat plate show little change or are nonspecific. A high index of suspicion is required and NOMI should be considered in those patients who develop unexplained clinical deterioration or failure to thrive while recovering from a cardiac event or major surgery.

DIAGNOSIS

Early diagnosis is critical to improving mortality or preventing the dire consequences of a short bowel syndrome secondary to massive small bowel infarction. Choosing the appropriate diagnostic studies at presentation, therefore, is essential as clinical deterioration is rapid and does not allow the luxury of multiple studies.

Angiography

Angiography remains the gold standard in AMI, allowing for diagnostic and therapeutic measures to address this condition. It has a high sensitivity (74% to 100%) and specificity (100%) with few complications.[4] Angiography must be biplanar. Lateral views provide optimal images of the origins of the major vessels, whereas anteroposterior views are best for visualizing the distal mesenteric vessels. Several studies have demonstrated increased survival in patients undergoing early angiography in AMI.[4,17] Whether angiogram is the preferred test in the face of peritoneal signs remains controversial. Some would favor immediate surgery in this setting, as signs of peritonitis indicate infarction. However, proponents of early angiography stress the importance of determining the cause, that is, embolic versus NOMI and providing a "roadmap" for the surgeon at laparotomy. Early angiography also allows for initiation of therapeutic maneuvers, as discussed later in this review.

Angiography is an invasive procedure and time consuming, often leading to substantial delays in time to surgery. Angiography may not be readily available in smaller community centers. Patients with significant hypovolemia or hypotension should not be considered for angiogram. Alternative approaches have been developed to address these concerns.

Multidetector CT Angiography

Multidetector CT angiography (MDCTA) is emerging as a new technology that may serve as an excellent alternative to angiography.[19,20] MDCTA is fast, noninvasive, and more readily available than angiography. Early on, results with a standard CT scan in AMI were variable, with a sensitivity of only 64% at best and often showing changes late in the course after the onset of bowel infarction. CT was of far more value in the evaluation of MVT. In a review of 72 patients with MVT, the investigators noted 100% sensitivity in acute cases, with 93% sensitivity in chronic MVT.[21] Findings included superior mesenteric vein thrombosis in association with bowel abnormalities such as thickening of the bowel wall. Therefore, in patients with suspected AMI, unless there is a prior history of deep venous thrombosis or a coagulation disorder, standard CT should not be the initial test of choice.

MDCTA, on the other hand, may provide valuable insight into the diagnosis of AMI and should be considered as an excellent initial study. Characteristic findings include mural thickening indicating the presence of mucosal edema, inflammation, or hemorrhage of the bowel wall.[22] Lack of mural enhancement reflects absence of mesenteric flow, which has a specificity approaching 100% for mesenteric ischemia. MDCTA allows direct visualization of vascular occlusion secondary to either arterial or venous thrombus. Emboli in the more distal branches may be difficult to see and, in this case, changes in the bowel wall may be the only diagnostic clue. In a prospective trial of 62 patients, 26 of whom had mesenteric ischemia, MDCTA was able to accurately diagnose all 26 patients.[23] Overall, combining vascular findings with the appearance of the bowel wall resulted in a specificity of 94% with a sensitivity of 96%. Advanced scanners with 3D imaging are becoming increasingly available which allows for a consistent approach. MDCTA does not provide the therapeutic options of visceral angiography, but may serve to stratify those patients who would be appropriate candidates for angiography versus those who should be taken directly to surgery.

Ultrasonography

Ultrasonography has a limited role in AMI. It may be technically difficult in patients presenting with ileus and bowel distention. It is incapable of seeing distal emboli and has little value in NOMI. In can detect proximal stenosis fairly accurately but cannot establish a diagnosis of mesenteric ischemia even in this setting, as these findings may be seen in asymptomatic individuals. For these reasons, ultrasonography is not recommended as an initial study in a disorder for which timing of the diagnosis is so critical.

Magnetic Resonance Angiography

Magnetic resonance angiography (MRA) also has limitations in its ability to detect NOMI or more distal occlusions. MRA is not universally available, is time consuming, and may delay therapeutic options. It is probably better used in the setting of CMI, as discussed later in this review.

TREATMENT

Because of the high mortality associated with AMI, early and aggressive treatment is warranted.

Initially patients need to be stabilized in terms of volume status and electrolyte abnormalities, with careful attention to intravascular volume loss as third spacing of fluids may be significant.

Broad-spectrum antibiotics should be initiated due to the high risk of bacterial translocation across the bowel wall in the ischemic segment. Causative factors should be addressed and modified if feasible, such as discontinuation of a vasoactive drug or initiation of anticoagulants in the setting of thrombosis. If the patient is not a candidate for angiography, glucagon can be administered intravenously to reduce vasospasm.[7] It should be given at 1 μg/kg/min and titrated up to 10 μg/kg/min as needed.

Early mesenteric angiography provides several therapeutic options. Following the diagnostic portion of the study, the catheter should be left in place for infusion of papaverine or other vasodilators. Papaverine is a phosphodiesterase inhibitor which has been shown to increase blood flow to marginally perfused tissue. The typical dose is 30 to 60 mg/h and can be maintained up to 5 days without complication. Other more specific therapeutic options otherwise will depend on the angiographic findings. If an embolus to the SMA is detected, thrombolytic agents may be infused directly into the embolus with excellent results.[24,25] The number of patients treated in this fashion remains small. In one series of 10 patients with an SMA embolus treated with 200,000 units of urokinase followed by a continuous infusion of 100,000 units/h, successful lysis of the embolus was achieved in nine patients (90%).[26] A review of the literature consisting mainly of case reports and small series found an overall success rate of 62.5% for thrombolytic therapy in patients with SMA emboli.[27] Contraindications to thombolysis relate primarily to risk of hemorrhage, as in patients with recent surgery or gastrointestinal bleed, patients with a recent stroke, or patients with an underlying clotting disorder. Hemorrhagic complications can usually be managed clinically, as normal coagulation parameters can be restored within hours of discontinuing the infusion. In the setting of peritoneal signs, the patient is better served by urgent laparotomy.

In patients with SMA embolus or thrombosis (**Fig. 1**), vasodilators have proven beneficial for treating splanchnic vasoconstriction, which occurs with AMI distal to

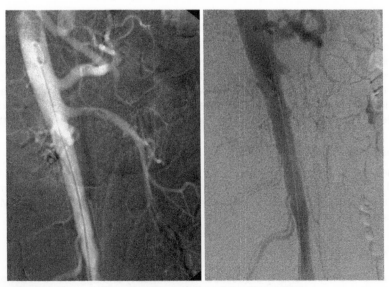

Fig. 1. SMA thrombosis (*left*); complete occlusion of the SMA (*right*).

the site of occlusion. As mentioned earlier, papaverine is effective in this setting. By reducing vasoconstriction, papaverine also lessens the risk of a reperfusion injury once the blood flow has been reestablished. This effect is manifested by a release of oxygen free radicals along with a local inflammatory response, which results in cytokine release and subsequent systemic effects on cardiac or renal function. Vasodilators are not to be considered an alternative to surgery, but used in conjunction with surgery to lessen the risk. Earlier studies have shown a substantial reduction in mortality associated with the use of papaverine from 70% to 90% to a lesser rate of 40% to 50%.

For NOMI the treatment is directed primarily at the underlying cause. As with other forms of intestinal ischemia, supportive care is essential. This care consists of intravenous fluids, broad spectrum antibiotics, and therapy directed at the underlying cardiac disease. Papaverine infused through an indwelling intra-arterial catheter may be adequate to treat the vasoconstriction without the need for surgery. The classic angiographic appearance in this setting is the "string of sausage" sign reflecting alternating dilatation and stenosis of the involved vessel. Serial angiograms should be followed until resolution of the vasospasm is confirmed. If at any time during the clinical course peritoneal signs develop, the patient should be taken to surgery. Other forms of therapy largely in the investigative phase include iloprost, a potent inhibitor of platelet aggregation and a fibrinolytic agent, rennin-angiotensin blockers, and free radical inhibitors. Few clinical data exist at this time to support their use.

MVT is also managed without surgery in those cases without evidence of progression to infarction. The management, in addition to supportive care as previously outlined, consists of the use of anticoagulants or thrombolytic therapy, or both. Intravenous heparin has been shown to decrease mortality from 59% to 22%, and rethrombosis from 26% to 14%. The use of thrombolytic agents has been limited to case reports only. Because these patients often have a persistent prothrombotic condition, long-term treatment with warfarin may be necessary. Thrombectomy should be reserved for those patients with an acute superior mesenteric vein or portal vein thrombosis.

SURGERY FOR AMI

Despite advances in diagnostic techniques and therapeutic options, surgery remains the treatment of choice in those patients with AMI who are operative candidates. At laparotomy, infarcted bowel is removed and blood flow is restored.[28] In patients found at laparotomy to have limited necrosis or indeterminate viability of the intestine, revascularization should always be performed first. Specific surgical techniques for revascularization are beyond the scope of this review. However, if the viability of the bowel remains in question at that point, then a "second look" procedure should be performed 24 to 48 hours later. Laparoscopy may be a less invasive alternative for the "second look" procedure. Postoperative mortality remains high, with the most common cause of death related to multisystem organ failure. Risk factors for increased mortality were assessed in a total of 72 patients undergoing surgery for AMI.[29] Independent predictors of mortality were age greater than 70 and delay in diagnosis (greater than 24 hours). Univariate analysis identified renal insufficiency, metabolic acidosis, symptom duration, and need for resection at "second look" procedure. These findings were confirmed in another review of 132 consecutive patients who underwent surgery for AMI.[30] Again it was age, time delay to surgery, shock, and metabolic acidosis which were identified as predictors of increased mortality. Cardiac disease, renal failure, and colonic disease were independent predictors. Surgery may offer the best opportunity for survival, but, as with other forms of therapy, a delay in diagnosis results in a poor outcome.

CHRONIC MESENTERIC ISCHEMIA

CMI is an uncommon form of mesenteric ischemia accounting for less than 5% of cases and virtually always seen in association with diffuse atherosclerosis (95%).[31] CMI presents most often with postprandial pain and significant weight loss accompanied often by postprandial diarrhea. Fear of eating is a direct consequence of the pain and accounts for the degree of weight loss, which is further accentuated by the development of malabsorption seen in up to 50% of cases. Nausea and vomiting may accompany the pain and in some cases be the dominant symptom. The pain occurs classically within 15 minutes of meal consumption and will last up to 1 to 3 hours. Chronic dull abdominal pain may develop in more advanced cases. As with AMI, the pain relates to an inadequate blood supply which is incapable of meeting the metabolic demands of the intestine which increase with meal intake.

In addition to atherosclerosis, CMI has also been associated with vascular occlusion secondary to fibromuscular dysplasia, Takayasu arteritis, vasculitis, radiation injury, or malignant encasement. Median arcuate ligament syndrome is a form of CMI caused by impingement of the celiac artery by the diaphragm. This syndrome is seen predominantly in women and is more commonly seen in younger patients presenting with unexplained abdominal pain and an abdominal bruit.

Patients with atherosclerosis and CMI are more commonly women (2:1) and most have major risk factors associated with atherosclerosis, such as hypertension, hyperlipidemia, or history of smoking. As a result, CMI rarely presents as an isolated finding, but frequently is seen in association with renal or cardiovascular disease. More than 90% of patients with CMI will have 2- or 3-vessel disease as the slow progression of atherosclerosis allows for the development of adequate collaterals. However the presence of mesenteric atherosclerosis alone does not establish the diagnosis. In a study of 553 asymptomatic elderly adults, 97 (17.5%) were found to have disease of the celiac or SMA.[32,33] Followed out to a mean of 6.5 years, there was no difference in mortality between those with mesenteric artery stenosis and those without. In a separate study, patients with asymptomatic, but more advanced, disease demonstrating greater than 50% occlusion in all 3 vessels followed out to 6 years, developed symptoms in 86% with a mortality rate of 40%.[34]

DIAGNOSIS
Ultrasound

Duplex ultrasonography with B-mode ultrasonography and Doppler waveform analysis serves as an excellent noninvasive means of accurately detecting mesenteric stenosis in CMI. It has a specificity of 92% to 100% for severe stenosis of the celiac or SMA but sensitivity is less at 70% to 89%. Established criteria for the diagnosis of severe stenosis rely on peak systolic velocity, exceeding 275 cm/s for the SMA and 200 cm/s for the celiac artery. Doppler ultrasonography remains a valuable initial screening tool.

Magnetic Resonance Angiography

MRA plays an important role in the early evaluation of patients suspected of having CMI. It is noninvasive and increasingly accurate. MRA was compared with angiography and surgery in a study of patients with significant stenosis of the splanchnic vessels, finding a sensitivity and specificity of 100% and 95%, respectively.[35] Its accuracy may relegate invasive angiography to a role in which catheter-based therapy is considered.

Mutidetector CT Angiography

As discussed earlier for AMI, MDCTA may be the procedure of choice for diagnosis of CMI, for essentially the same reasons. It is noninvasive, rapid, and may offer a more complete examination than conventional angiography. MDCTA images distal segments more effectively, and can outline the vascular narrowing and the atherosclerotic plaque itself.[3] MDCTA therefore should be considered as a first line alternative to angiography for diagnostic purposes.

Visible Light Spectroscopy

Visible light spectroscopy is an endoscopic technique that can measure mucosal perfusion in the gastrointestinal tract. It relies on the delivery of white light by a fiberoptic probe to measure the percent saturation of hemoglobin in the mucosal capillary network. This measure directly reflects perfusion. In a small trial of 33 patients, three of whom had proven CMI, the technique distinguished all three with CMI from the healthy controls and showed significant improvement in the same patients after revascularization.[36]

Angiography

The advantage of angiography in CMI is the ability to therapeutically intervene, possibly avoiding major surgery in those who may not be ideal surgical candidates. The development of stents has significantly improved the long-term efficacy of this procedure (**Fig. 2**). A review of recent studies reports a procedural success rate of

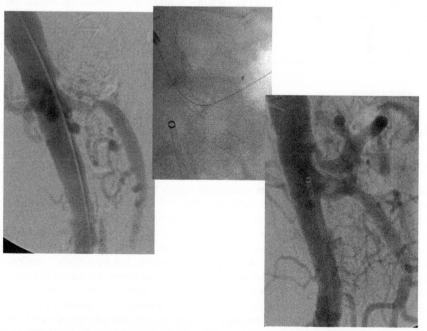

Fig. 2. Celiac occlusion and SMA stenosis (*left*); stents in celiac and SMA (*center*); celiac improved and SMA wide open (*right*).

88% to 100%, with initial relief of symptoms in 82% to 100%.[37] Long-term success was evaluated in a single institution review of percutaneous intervention in 31 patients with symptomatic CMI.[38] All patients in the study had three-vessel disease with a median of two-vessel occlusion on angiography. Eighty-six percent had 1 vessel treated and the remainder had two vessels treated. Overall 90-day mortality was 20% with major morbidity in 6%. At 1 year 70% were asymptomatic and at 5 years it was only 56%. Restenosis occurred in 20% of vessels at a median of 0.29 years, and primary patency rate at 7 years was 69%. In 50% of these patients reintervention was possible with resolution of their symptoms.

Surgery

Surgery remains the most effective long-term treatment of CMI and can be performed electively in most cases with reduced morbidity and mortality. The surgery most often involves endarterectomy or vascular bypass. In three large series of surgical revascularization in patients with symptomatic CMI, 5-year survival averaged 63% to 71% and 5-year patency rates averaged 78% to 92%.[28]

Compared with percutaneous intervention, long-term patency rates for surgery are superior, yet early morbidity and mortality are increased.[39] In a direct comparison of outcomes, 49 patients with CMI underwent either surgical revascularization (26 patients) or endovascular repair (23 patients).[40] Patients were well matched in this retrospective review. Overall 30-day mortality in the surgical group (SG) was 8% compared with 0% for patients undergoing endovascular treatment (ET). However, initial relief from symptoms in the SG was 100% versus 90% for ET with long-term (24.7 months) relief in 89% versus 75%, respectively. Restenosis and recurrence of symptoms was more common with ET than in the SG, 25% and 9% versus 8% and 0%, respectively. Morbidity early on and mortality at the end of follow-up were higher in the SG than with ET, 42% and 31% versus 4% and 4%, respectively. Similar findings were demonstrated in a separate study, yet there was no difference seen in immediate morbidity or mortality between patients undergoing surgery or endovascular revascularization.[41] Overall this favors surgery, reserving endovascular revascularization for those patients with excessive comorbidities.

ISCHEMIC COLITIS

It is difficult to determine the true incidence of ischemic colitis (IC) in the elderly population, as so often cases go undiagnosed or are frequently misdiagnosed as acute infectious diarrhea or inflammatory bowel disease. Yet it does represent the most common type of mesenteric ischemia and incidence rates for IC range from 6.1 to 47 per 100,000 person-years.[42] Several factors predispose the colon to ischemic injury. Typically the colon receives less blood supply than the rest of the gastrointestinal tract, and the microvascular network within the colon is less well developed.[43] Also there are two classic "watershed" areas in the splenic flexure and restosigmoid, as previously described, which are particularly vulnerable to an ischemic injury. IC is generally considered a nonocclusive form of ischemia, and causative factors are those associated with a low-flow state. As a result, risk factors are essentially identical to those previously discussed with NOMI. However in most cases the cause is speculative, as the inciting event has resolved by the time of presentation. In a review of IC following MI, IC was found to be the most common endoscopic diagnosis made after MI in patients undergoing sigmoidoscopy or colonoscopy, and was found in 0.13% of MI patients.[44] Following major vascular surgery the incidence was somewhat higher at 0.6% to 3.1%, but, in those cases, mortality approached 67%.[45] The investigators stressed the importance of early recognition and preventative measures, such as avoidance of systemic vasopressors and strict attention to intravascular pressure and volume status.

IC represents a broad spectrum of clinical disorders ranging from benign reversible colitis to fulminant ischemic necrosis. Fortunately most cases do follow a benign course, but predicting at onset which patients will progress may be difficult. In a retrospective review of 73 patients with IC, risk factors for more aggressive disease were identified.[46] In a univariate analysis, six risk factors were identified, including age younger than 80, male sex, fever greater than 38°C, abdominal tenderness, absence of lower intestinal bleeding, and low bicarbonate levels. In multivariate analysis all but fever and low bicarbonate level remained significant. A second study supported these findings in 129 patients, also demonstrating a worse prognosis in those with limited right-sided colitis.[47]

IC should be considered in any elderly person presenting with acute onset of lower abdominal, crampy pain associated with urgent bloody stools. Physical examination may reveal abdominal tenderness, often reflecting the location of the involved segment. The laboratory results are nonspecific, only showing diagnostic changes of acidosis or elevated lactic acid late in the course of the disease. More common aspects of the differential diagnosis are often considered first, such as infectious colitis, pseudomembranous colitis, diverticulitis, inflammatory bowel disease, or colon cancer, which may further delay the diagnosis.

Because these patients are elderly with multiple comorbidities, aggressive supportive care at the onset is essential. These measures are outlined in the section on AMI. An effort should be made to identify and correct the inciting event if evident. Stools should be sent for bacterial cultures (including *Escherichia coli* O157:H7), *Clostridium difficile* toxin, and ova and parasites. The plain film of the abdomen offers little early on and has largely been supplanted by the CT scan, which offers significantly more information regarding location of disease and degree of involvement. Although rarely diagnostic, segmental involvement is the most common form of presentation, seen in 89% of patients presenting with CI. There is little need for angiography in the evaluation of CI. Blood flow has usually returned to normal by the time the patient becomes symptomatic, and findings on angiogram rarely correlate with symptoms of CI in the elderly.[42] Colonoscopy can be safely performed in most patients with CI and has become the preferred diagnostic test. Characteristic findings include a segmental colitis which may progress from submucosal hemorrhage to nonspecific acute inflammation, ulceration, and submucosal sloughing.

Treatment of CI generally consists of supportive care as outlined, with broad spectrum antibiotics in moderate to severe disease. Fortunately most cases are self-limited and require no more specific therapy. Surgery plays a role in those patients with peritoneal signs, or evidence of severe disease with infarction or perforation. Massive bleeding may rarely occur which requires segmental resection. Long-term complications of stricture formation may also require resection if clinically symptomatic. There exists a small subset of patients who develop a form of chronic IC which persists for several months beyond their initial presentation. These patients do not respond to therapy directed to reducing inflammation, and may also come to segmental resection. As less than 5% of patients with CI recur, resection in this setting is generally curative.

SUMMARY

Mesenteric ischemia in the elderly is an uncommon but often fatal disorder for which the prognosis depends entirely on the speed and accuracy of the diagnosis. A high index of suspicion is required as the early signs and symptoms, at a time when ischemic changes are reversible, are typically nonspecific or absent. Pain out of proportion to the physical examination, or clinical deterioration in the postoperative setting should alert the clinician to this possibility. For AMI, surgery still remains the best hope for recovery, but in CMI, percutaneous revascularization may play an increasingly important role. The most common form of mesenteric ischemia is CI, which, fortunately, in most cases requires no specific therapy other than supportive care.

REFERENCES

1. Herbert GS, Steele SR. Acute and chronic mesenteric ischemia. Surg Clin North Am 2007;87:1115–34.
2. Greenwald DA, Brandt LJ, Reinus JF. Ischemic bowel disease in the elderly. Gastroenterol Clin North Am 2001;30(2):445–73.
3. Ozden N, Gurses B. Mesenteric ischemia in the elderly. Clin Geriatr Med 2007;23:871–87.
4. Brandt LJ, Boley SJ. AGA technical review on intestinal ischemia. Gastroenterology 2000;118:954–68.
5. Burns BJ, Brandt LJ. Intestinal ischemia. Gastroenterol Clin North Am 2003;32(4):1127–43.
6. Chang W, Chang J, Longo W. Update in management of mesenteric ischemia. World J Gastroenterol 2006;12(20):3243–7.
7. Oldenburg WA, Lau LL, Rodenberg TJ, et al. Acute mesenteric ischemia: a clinical review. Arch Intern Med 2004;164:1054–62.
8. Mamode N, Pickford I, Lieberman P. Failure to improve outcome in acute mesenteric ischemia: seven year review. Eur J Surg 1999;165(3):203–8.
9. Acosta S, Ogren M, Sternby NH, et al. Incidence of acute thrombo-embolic occlusion of the superior mesenteric artery: a population based study. Eur J Vasc Endovasc Surg 2004;27(2):145–50.
10. Bartone G, Severino BU, Armellino MT, et al. Clinical symptoms of intestinal vascular disorders. Radiol Clin North Am 2008;46:887–9.
11. Lobo Martinez E, Carvajosa E, Sacco O, et al. Embolectomy in mesenteric ischemia. Rev Esp Enferm Dig 1993;83:351–4.
12. Lyon C, Clark DC. Diagnosis of acute abdominal pain in older patients. Am Fam Physician 2006;74:1537–44.
13. Pique JM. Management of gut ischemia. Indian J Gastroenterol 2006;25(Suppl):S39–42.
14. Ritz JP, Runkel N, Berger G, et al. Prognostic factors in mesenteric ischemia. Zen Chir 1997;122:332–8 [German].
15. Acosta S, Ogren M, Sternby NH, et al. Clinical implications for the management of acute thromboemolic occlusion of the superior mesenteric artery. Ann Surg 2005;241(3):516–22.
16. Martinez JR, Hogan GJ. Mesenteric ischemia. Emerg Med Clin North Am 2004;22:909–28.
17. Berland T, Oldenburg WA. Acute mesenteric ischemia. Curr Gastroenterol Rep 2008;10:341–6.
18. Acosta S, Ogren M, Sternby NH, et al. Fatal nonocclusive mesenteric ischaemia: population-based incidence and risk factors. J Intern Med 2006;259:305–13.
19. Romano S, Niola R, Maglione F, et al. Small bowel vascular disorders from arterial etiology and impaired venous drainage. Radiol Clin North Am 2008;46:891–908.

20. Horton KM, Fishman EK. Multidetector CT angiography in the diagnosis of mesenteric ischemia. Radiol Clin North Am 2007;45:275–88.
21. Rhee RY, Gloviczki P, Mendonca CT, et al. Mesenteric venous thrombosis: still a lethal disease in the 1990s. J Vasc Surg 1994;20:688–97.
22. Levy AD. Mesenteric ischemia. Radiol Clin North Am 2007;45:593–9.
23. Kirkpatrick ID, Kroeker MA, Greenberg HM. Biphasic CT with mesenteric CT angiography in the evaluation of acute mesenteric ischemia: initial experience. Radiology 2003;229(1):91–8.
24. Kozuch PL, Brandt LJ. Review article: diagnosis and management of mesenteric ischaemia with an emphasis on pharmacotherapy. Aliment Pharmacol Ther 2005; 21:201–15.
25. Frishman WH, Novak S, Brandt LJ, et al. Pharmacologic management of mesenteric occlusive disease. Cardiol Rev 2008;16:59–68.
26. Simo G, Echenagusia AJ, Camunez F, et al. Superior mesenteric embolism: local fibronolytic treatment with urokinase. Radiology 1997;204:775–9.
27. Shoots IG, Levi NM, Reekers JA, et al. Thrombolytic therapy for acute superior mesenteric artery occlusion. J Vasc Interv Radiol 2005;16:317–29.
28. Wain RA, Hines G. Surgical management of mesenteric occlusive disease: a contemporary review of invasive and minimally invasive techniques. Cardiol Rev 2008;16:69–75.
29. Kougias P, Lau D, El Sayed H, et al. Determinants of mortality and treatment outcome following surgical interventions for acute mesenteric ischemia. J Vasc Surg 2007;46:467–74.
30. Acosta-Merida MA, Marchena-Gomez J, Hemmersbach-Miller M, et al. Identification of risk factors for perioperative mortality in acute mesenteric ischemia. World J Surg 2006;30:1579–85.
31. Sreenarashimhaiah J. Chronic mesenteric ischemia. Best Pract Res Clin Gastroenterol 2005;19(2):283–95.
32. Wilson DB, Mostafavi K, Craven TE, et al. Clinical course of mesenteric artery stenosis in elderly Americans. Arch Intern Med 2006;166:2095–100.
33. Hansen KJ, Wilson DB, Craven TE, et al. Mesenteric artery disease in the elderly. J Vasc Surg 2004;40:45–52.
34. Thomas JH, Blake K, Pierce GE, et al. The clinical course of asymptomatic mesenteric arterial stenosis. J Vasc Surg 1998;27(5):840–4.
35. Meaney JF, Prince MR, Nostrant TT, et al. Gadolinium – enhanced MR angiography of visceral arteries in patients with suspected chronic mesenteric ischemia. J Magn Reson Imaging 1997;1:171–6.
36. Friedland S, Benaron D, Coogan S, et al. Diagnosis of chronic mesenteric ischemia by visible light spectroscopy during endoscopy. Gastrointest Endosc 2007;65(2):294–300.
37. Soga Y, Yokoi H, Iwabuchi M, et al. Endovascular treatment of chronic mesenteric ischemia. Circ J 2008;72:1198–200.
38. Lee RW, Bakken AM, Palchik E, et al. Long-term outcomes of endoluminal therapy for chronic atherosclerotic occlusive mesenteric disease. Ann Vasc Surg 2008;11:541–6.
39. Kruger AJ, Walker PJ, Foster WJ, et al. Open surgery for atherosclerotic chronic mesenteric ischemia. J Vasc Surg 2007;46:941–5.
40. Biebl M, Oldenburg WA, Paz-Fumagalli R, et al. Surgical and interventional visceral revascularization for the treatment of chronic mesenteric ischemia – when to prefer which? World J Surg 2007;31:562–8.

41. Atkins MD, Kwolek CJ, LaMuraglia GM, et al. Surgical revascularization versus endovascular therapy for chronic mesenteric ischemia: a comparative experience. J Vasc Surg 2007;45:1162–7.
42. Brandt LJ. Bloody diarrhea in an elderly patient. Gastroenterology 2005;128: 157–63.
43. Taourel P, Aufort S, Merigeaud S, et al. Imaging of ischemic colitis. Radiol Clin North Am 2008;46:909–24.
44. Cappell MS, Mahajan D, Kurupath V. Characterization of ischemic colitis associated with myocardial infarction: an analysis of 23 patients. Am J Med 2006;119: 527.e1–9.
45. Steele SR. Ischemic colitis complicating major vascular surgery. Surg Clin North Am 2007;878:1099–114.
46. Huguier M, Barrier A, Boelle PY, et al. Ischemic colitis. Am J Surg 2006;192: 679–84.
47. Scharff JR, Longo WE, Vartanian SM, et al. Ischemic colitis: spectrum of disease and outcome. Surgery 2003;134:624–30.

Solitary Rectal Ulcer Syndrome and Stercoral Ulcers

Yair Edden, MD, Shirley S. Shih, MD, Steven D. Wexner, MD*

KEYWORDS

• Rectal ulcer • Stercoral ulcers • Solitary rectal ulcer syndrome

Colonic ulcerations can affect the entire colon and rectum. These ulcerations have variable clinical presentation according to the anatomic location and underlying pathology. Diverse etiologies may lead to colonic ulceration, for example, inflammatory bowel diseases, oral drugs (mostly nonsteroidal anti-inflammatory drugs [NSAIDs]), local or diffuse ischemia, and different intestinal microorganisms. An ulcer may also herald a concealed malignant disease. In most cases, colonic ulceration is associated with diffuse colitis in the acute setup or with inflammatory bowel diseases, and to a lesser extent the ulceration is defined as solitary. This article focuses on two of the less commonly diagnosed diseases: solitary rectal ulcer syndrome and stercoral ulceration, both related to local tissue ischemia and often seen in the elderly population.

SOLITARY RECTAL ULCER SYNDROME

Solitary rectal ulcer syndrome (SRUS), as the name implies, consists of several different clinical pathologic processes. These processes, however, end in a mutual common pathway that is associated with reduced blood perfusion of the rectal mucosa, leading to local ischemia and ulceration. SRUS was described in the early nineteenth century by the French anatomist J. Cruvilhier in his report on chronic rectal ulcer.[1] However, the distinctive histopathologic characteristics were defined in 1969 by Madigan and Morson.[2] SRUS is a rare syndrome with a prevalence of less than 1 in 100,000 per year. The current literature comprises case series studies and sporadic case reports.[3–8]

Clinical Presentation

Due to its rarity, nonspecific signs, and symptoms and various causes, SRUS diagnosis is delayed in many cases. However, chronic constipation, strenuous defecation,

Department of Colorectal Surgery, Cleveland Clinic, 2950 Cleveland Clinic Boulevard, Weston, FL 33331, USA
* Corresponding author.
E-mail address: deanh@ccf.org (S.D. Wexner).

Gastroenterol Clin N Am 38 (2009) 541–545
doi:10.1016/j.gtc.2009.06.010
0889-8553/09/$ – see front matter © 2009 Elsevier Inc. All rights reserved.

bloody and mucous secretions per rectum, and nonspecific pelvic pain are the major complaints encountered by physicians.[3,8,9]

Diagnosis

In many cases the initial clinical workup includes endoscopic visualization of the colon, revealing a solitary ulcer on the anterior rectal wall from which biopsies should be taken to rule out a malignant disease. Despite the diverse causes the microscopic changes are analogous, comprising fibromuscular obliteration and disorientation of the muscularis mucosa (**Fig. 1**).[2]

Etiology

As mentioned earlier, the underlying cause for this type of ulceration is chronic local ischemia of the colonic wall. Although the gradual sequence of this pathology may originate for various reasons, SRUS has been related to several independent clinical settings.

Rectal prolapse and intussusception
Rectal intussusception, which may lead to full-thickness rectal prolapse, results in localized vascular trauma and ischemia, initiating solitary local ulceration.[3,8,10]

Paradoxic contraction of the pelvic floor muscles
This uncoordinated sequence of muscle contraction and relaxation required for the defecation process, also called puborectalis syndrome or pelvic outlet obstruction, causes increased pressure inside the rectum and anal canal, generating ischemia and ulceration.[8,11]

Trauma
Localized rectal trauma, mainly from digitation or self-instrumentation, has been proposed as one of the causes of SRUS. Supportive evidence for anal intercourse as a basis for rectal ulceration do exist; however, conflicting conclusions have been published as well.[12,13]

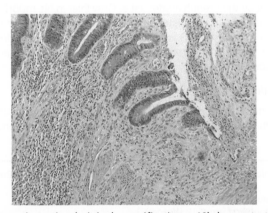

Fig. 1. Hematoxylin-eosin section (original magnification, ×10) demonstrating the histologic features typical of solitary rectal ulcer including surface ulceration, reactive epithelial changes, and fibromuscular hyperplasia of the lamina propria. (*Courtesy of* Y.E. Johnston, MD, M.E. Berho, MD, Department of Pathology, Cleveland Clinic, Weston, FL.)

Extraneous defecation due to chronic constipation and hard stool mimics the pathogenesis of outlet obstruction when high pressure chronically reduces the mucosal blood flow in the rectum aside from local mechanical-induced tears.[3,14]

Radiotherapy and ergotamine suppositories

Further supportive evidence for the substantial role of mucosal perfusion and ischemia in the pathogenesis of SRUS is the use of ergotamine suppositories. These strong vasoconstrictors, indicated for treating severe migraine, have been shown to induce local ischemia and ulceration. Radiotherapy, which in the long term affects permanently small blood vessels, has been cited as potentially antecedent to SRUS as well.[15,16]

Treatment

Because the etiology of SRUS is diverse, the therapeutic approach is variable. After the diagnosis is reached, usually by direct endoscopy and pathology results from biopsies that ruled out malignancy, the next diagnostic step is detecting the underlying pathologic basis of disease. Thorough history-taking to rule out local trauma or behavioral patterns and how to avoid these may be the initial treatment. Further imaging and physiologic studies are usually indicated, including rectal ultrasound, cinedefecography, and contrast enema. These procedures indicate muscle relaxation-related pathologies as well as other mechanical disorders.

Local treatments with steroid or sulfasalazine enemas were not effective in all patients,[9] whereas using a fibrin sealant achieved good results in six patients followed for 1 year.[17] For some underlying pathologies conservative measures such as stool softeners, adequate daily water intake, and cessation of digitation, or stopping the use of relevant suppositories address the clinical signs and symptoms. However, when pelvic outlet obstruction is the source of local ischemia the therapeutic aspects should focus on biofeedback training sessions, educating the patient to control the proper muscle contraction and relaxation sequence.[3,8,9]

In some cases when rectal prolapse is diagnosed, surgical intervention is indicated. Choosing the correct surgery, which may vary from a resection using the perineal approach to abdominal operation or even a permanent colostomy, should be made independently for each patient.[9]

Outcomes

Depending on the underlying cause and the chosen treatment, the therapeutic outcomes varies. Several studies of a low volume of patients and short follow-up, describe the outcome of different solutions for patients diagnosed with SRUS. When seven patients were treated by biofeedback alone for symptomatic puborectalis syndrome, an improvement in the symptoms was noted with a follow-up of 6 months. In another series of 13 patients, improvement was documented on clinical symptoms and on quality of life. However, among the 9 patients examined after the treatment the ulceration did not heal completely.[18] Sitzler and colleagues[19] reported the long-term surgical outcomes of 66 patients who underwent 72 procedures for SRUS. This study revealed improvement among 52% of the patients who did not have a colostomy.

Conclusions

SRUS is the final clinical outcome of different pathologic settings associated with compromised perfusion to the rectal mucosa. Identifying the correct foundation allows proper treatment with optimal results.

STERCORAL ULCERATION AND PERFORATION

Large bowel perforation is a surgical emergency and requires the utmost attention. Due its copious bacterial flora, outflow of large bowel content results in peritonitis and sepsis that leads to significant morbidity and mortality if left unattended. In many cases expeditious surgical intervention is indicated.

Stercoral perforation, a tear of the colonic wall due to localized intraluminal pressure induced by an outsized, hard stool is considered rare because less than 100 cases have been described in the modern literature have been described since 1965, although additional unreported cases should be assumed.[3,20,21]

Hard stool consequential of chronic and severe constipation pressing constantly against a particular area of the bowel wall causes localized ischemia which, if prolonged, may induce rectal bleeding and develop into necrosis and perforation, followed by purulent and fecal peritonitis.

The cause of stercoral ulceration originates in severe chronic constipation of varying pathology, leading to a large volume of stool that hardens over time. Eventually a single location along the large bowel, usually in the sigmoid colon, is subjected to ischemia, ulceration, necrosis, and perforation.[22,23] In most of the cases reported in the literature, the perforation occurs in the sigmoid colon.[3] This is the narrowest part of the colon where the water content of intraluminal contents has been absorbed to the maximum, so the stool is in its most solid form. However, reports of perforation in different anatomic locations have been described.[22] The clinical presentation of stercoral ulceration is nonspecific: lower abdominal pain and rectal bleeding associated with constipation are common, and could be attributed to several other underlying pathologies. For this reason in many cases the presenting scenario of a stercoral ulcer is a perforation leading to emergent surgery with high morbidity and mortality. As with many pathologies, prevention is the optimal treatment and the population at high risk should be addressed properly.

Constipation among the elderly population is common and due to various reasons, and each case should be evaluated separately.[24] It is important to bear in mind that in some cases severe constipation has a lethal outcome.

REFERENCES

1. Cruveilhier J. Ulcere chronique du rectum. Anatomie pathologique du corps humain. Paris: JB Bailliere; 1829.
2. Madigan MR, Morson BC. Solitary ulcer of the rectum. Gut 1969;10(11):871–81.
3. Nagar AB. Isolated colonic ulcers: diagnosis and management. Curr Gastroenterol Rep 2007;9(5):422–8.
4. Ortega AE, Klipfel N, Kelso R, et al. Changing concepts in the pathogenesis, evaluation, and management of solitary rectal ulcer syndrome. Am Surg 2008;74(10): 967–72.
5. Meurette G, Siproudhis L, Regenet N, et al. Poor symptomatic relief and quality of life in patients treated for "solitary rectal ulcer syndrome without external rectal prolapse". Int J Colorectal Dis 2008;23(5):521–6.
6. Marchal F, Bresler L, Brunaud L, et al. Solitary rectal ulcer syndrome: a series of 13 patients operated with a mean follow-up of 4.5 years. Int J Colorectal Dis 2001; 16(4):228–33.
7. Royes CA, Williams NP, Hanchard B, et al. Solitary rectal ulcer syndrome. West Indian Med J 1992;41(4):152–5.
8. Vaizey CJ, van den Bogaerde JB, Emmanuel AV, et al. Solitary rectal ulcer syndrome. Br J Surg 1998;85(12):1617–23.

9. Torres C, Khaikin M, Bracho J, et al. Solitary rectal ulcer syndrome: clinical findings, surgical treatment, and outcomes. Int J Colorectal Dis 2007;22(11): 1389–93.

10. Felt-Bersma RJ, Stella MT, Cuesta MA. Rectal prolapse, rectal intussusception, rectocele, solitary rectal ulcer syndrome, and enterocele. Gastroenterol Clin North Am 2008;37(3):645–68.

11. Morio O, Meurette G, Desfourneaux V, et al. Anorectal physiology in solitary ulcer syndrome: a case-matched series. Dis Colon Rectum 2005;48(10):1917–22.

12. Rutter KR, Riddell RH. The solitary ulcer syndrome of the rectum. Clin Gastroenterol 1975;4(3):505–30.

13. Contractor TQ, Contractor QQ. Traumatic solitary rectal ulcer in Saudi Arabia. A distinct entity? J Clin Gastroenterol 1995;21(4):298–300.

14. Chong VH, Jalihal A. Solitary rectal ulcer syndrome: characteristics, outcomes and predictive profiles for persistent bleeding per rectum. Singapore Med J 2006;47(12):1063–8.

15. Eckardt VF, Kanzler G, Remmele W. Anorectal ergotism: another cause of solitary rectal ulcers. Gastroenterology 1986;91(5):1123–7.

16. Pfeifer J, Reissman P, Wexner SD. Ergotamine induced complex rectovaginal fistula: report of a case. Dis Colon Rectum 1995;38:1224–6.

17. Ederle A, Bulighin G, Orlandi PG, et al. Endoscopic application of human fibrin sealant in the treatment of solitary rectal ulcer syndrome. Endoscopy 1992; 24(8):736–7.

18. Vaizey CJ, Roy AJ, Kamm MA. Prospective evaluation of the treatment of solitary rectal ulcer syndrome with biofeedback. Gut 1997;41(6):817–20.

19. Sitzler PJ, Kamm MA, Nicholls RJ, et al. Long-term clinical outcome of surgery for solitary rectal ulcer syndrome. Br J Surg 1998;85(9):1246–50.

20. Tokunaga Y, Hata K, Nishitai R, et al. Spontaneous perforation of the rectum with possible stercoral etiology: report of a case and review of the literature. Surg Today 1998;28(9):937–9.

21. Serpell JW, Nicholls RJ. Stercoral perforation of the colon. Br J Surg 1990;77(12): 1325–9.

22. Dubinsky I. Stercoral perforation of the colon: case report and review of the literature. J Emerg Med 1996;14(3):323–5.

23. Lui RC, Herz B, Plantilla E, et al. Stercoral perforation of the colon: report of a new location. Am J Gastroenterol 1988;83(4):457–9.

24. McCrea GL, Miaskowski C, Stotts NA, et al. Pathophysiology of constipation in the older adult. World J Gastroenterol 2008;14(17):2631–8.

Pharmacologic Consideration of Commonly Used Gastrointestinal Drugs in the Elderly

Barbara J. Zarowitz, PharmD, BCPS, CGP[a,b]

KEYWORDS

- Drug-induced conditions • Gastrointestinal • Medications
- Aged • Proton pump inhibitors • Antinauseants • Laxatives

Gastrointestinal (GI) manifestations in older adults can be caused or alleviated by drug therapy. GI medications, such as proton pump inhibitors and histamine-2 receptor antagonists, are among the most commonly used medications in long-term care facilities in the United States.[1] As in most other areas of medicine, evidence-based approaches are advocated when clinicians select medications to mitigate or treat GI conditions and prevent drug-induced GI adverse events. Assessment of the risk versus benefit of treatment in frail elderly patients is complex because of underlying pathophysiologic changes and responses to drug therapy as well as changes in drug metabolism or elimination. In addition, the literature is replete with information on younger populations but clinicians are frequently faced with assessing whether results of trials performed in younger adults can be applied to the care of older Americans. This article reviews the alterations in pharmacokinetic disposition of medications that occur with aging and highlights the pharmacology of commonly used GI drugs. Selected GI conditions that are drug-induced and preventable are identified, and recommendations for GI drugs to be avoided in older adults are provided.

PHARMACOKINETIC CHANGES OF AGING AND RESULTING PHARMACODYNAMIC RESPONSE
Absorption

Physiologic changes of the GI tract with aging include increased gastric pH, delayed gastric emptying, reduced GI blood flow, and slowed intestinal transit.[2] As a result of these changes, older persons can be expected to exhibit decreased bioavailability of

[a] Professional Services, Omnicare, Inc., 13975 Farmington Road, Livonia, MI 48150, USA
[b] College of Pharmacy and Health Sciences, Wayne State University, Detroit, MI 48201, USA
E-mail address: barbara.zarowitz@omnicare.com

Gastroenterol Clin N Am 38 (2009) 547–562
doi:10.1016/j.gtc.2009.06.011
0889-8553/09/$ – see front matter © 2009 Elsevier Inc. All rights reserved.

gastro.theclinics.com

medications with acid-dependent absorption, such as iron, and slowed absorption of medications, especially those that are enteric-coated.[2]

Metabolism: First Pass

There is a 20% to 30% reduction in liver mass and hepatic blood flow with advancing age but perfusion of individual hepatocytes remains constant.[2] Drug metabolism that depends on hepatic blood flow can be reduced in older persons. Changes in drug absorption with aging have been attributed to alterations in the metabolism of medications during their first pass through the liver, known as first pass metabolism.[3] For example, morphine clearance is reduced about 33% in older persons leading to longer half-lives and the need for lower oral doses. The average clearance of propranolol declines, whereas the oral bioavailability increases. In the elderly there is a doubling of the bioavailability of chlormethiazole, lidocaine, labetalol, verapamil, propranolol, and levodopa.[3] The practical consequences of alterations in drug absorption, bioavailability, and first pass metabolism result in the need to start with lower doses and perhaps longer dosing intervals between doses to avoid the risk of drug accumulation and toxicity.

Metabolism: Elimination

The effects of aging of the liver drug metabolizing enzymes are less clear. Activity of the cytochrome (CYP) P450 isoenzymes, 1A2, 2C9, 2C19, 2E1, and 3A4, may be decreased but do not universally result in reduced clearance of substrates for those enzymes. Variation in CYP function may be more related to changes in lifestyle and disease-related hepatic dysfunction than to aging.[2] Drug metabolism by conjugation with glucuronic acid or oxidation is typically preserved with aging. As a result, studies of oxazepam, lorazepam, and temazepam have not identified changes in drug pharmacokinetics in older persons.[2]

Renal Elimination

Renal function progressively declines with age independent of the development of any renal disease. By the age of 85 years the average creatinine clearance (ClCr) has declined to 50% of what it was at 25 years of age.[2] The Baltimore Longitudinal Study of Aging prospectively found a decrease in ClCr of 0.75 mL/min/y.[4] Most important is the potential to under recognize the decline in renal function when evaluating serum creatinine, soley.[5] As a result of decreased production of creatinine with decreasing mobility and lower muscle mass in frail elderly individuals, serum creatinine can appear normal despite significant reductions in glomerular filtration rate (GFR) or ClCr.[6–8] As a result, renal function should be estimated using either the modification in Diet for Renal Disease (MDRD) or Cockcroft and Gault equations for GFR or ClCr, respectively. Most clinical laboratories calculate GFR by MDRD whenever a serum creatinine is analyzed. Clinical pharmacists routinely use the Cockcroft and Gault equation to estimate ClCr for dosing of renal elimination of medications.

Older persons are subject to compromises in renal function secondary to progression of chronic conditions such as diabetes and hypertension.[5] Hanlon and colleagues[9] have published an extensive list of medications affected by renal impairment with recommendations for dosage reduction or avoidance. Among GI medications, ranitidine and cimetidine were recommended for dosage reduction in persons with ClCr less than 50 mL/min. The manufacturer recommends a 50% reduction in the dose of metoclopramide in patients with ClCr less than 40 mL/min.[10]

PHARMACOLOGY OF COMMONLY USED GI MEDICATIONS

Table 1 lists agents used commonly in older persons with GI conditions. A brief review of the pharmacokinetic and pharmacodynamic effects, significant drug interactions, side effects, and considerations unique to the elderly is provided.

Proton Pump Inhibitors

Proton pump inhibitors are generally considered safe and effective in older persons.[11] Common adverse effects include headache, diarrhea, nausea, flatulence, and abdominal cramps.[10,11] More serious consequences can occur with long-term administration of proton pump inhibitors. In a matched case-control study, patients older than 50 years of age who take proton pump inhibitors for more than 1 year were found to be at increased risk of hip fracture and the effect is dose-related.[12] The investigators found that high-dose proton pump inhibitor therapy in long-term users increased the risk for hip fracture compared with nonusers (95% confidence interval [CI] 1.80–3.9, $P<.001$), perhaps as a result of reduced absorption of calcium. The lowest effective dose of proton pump inhibitors is recommended in older persons. Proton pump inhibitors have been associated with causing diarrhea induced by *Clostridium difficile* and should only be prescribed in individuals with a clear indication and for the shortest possible duration.[13]

There is a clear relationship between drug exposure and the pharmacodynamic response (ie, gastric acid suppression, healing) to proton pump inhibitors.[14] Proton pump inhibitors are absorbed well and should be taken approximately 1 hour before

Table 1
Medications commonly used to manage GI conditions

Condition	Medication(s) Class
GERD, NERD, peptic ulcer disease, *H pylori*	Proton pump inhibitors: omeprazole, lansoprazole, pantoprazole, rabeprazole, esomeprazole, and dexlansoprazole Histamine-2 receptor antagonists: cimetidine, ranitidine, famotidine, and nizatidine Metoclopramide, bismuth subsalicylate
Constipation	Bulk-forming: psyllium, methylcellulose, polycarbophil Osmotic: lactulose, polyethylene glycol, sorbitol Emollient: docusate, mineral oil Saline cathartic: magnesium citrate, MOM, sodium phosphate Stimulant: bisacodyl, senna Chloride channel activator: lubiprostone Opioid receptor antagonist: methylnatrexone Selective serotonin partial agonist: tegaserod
Nausea and vomiting	Phenothiazines: prochlorperazine, promethazine Corticosteroids: dexamethasone Anticholinergics: scopolamine, hyoscyamine 5-HT$_3$ antagonists: ondansetron, granisetron, dolasetron Dopamine agonists: metoclopramide
Diarrhea	Bismuth subsalicylate, diphenoxylate, loperamide, octreotide
Antispasmodics	Hyoscyamine, atropine, dicyclomine, propantheline, chlordiazepoxide

Abbreviations: 5-HT$_3$, 5-hydroxytryptamine 3 receptor; GERD, gastroesophageal reflux disease; MOM, magnesium hydroxide; NERD, nonerosive reflux disease.
Data from Refs.[10,11,14,17,19,21,26,30]

eating.[14] Furthermore, because they are acid labile, proton pump inhibitors are manufactured as either enteric-coated granules within a capsule or enteric-coated tablets to inhibit degradation by gastric acid. Formulations should not be crushed or chewed before administration.[10] A rapid-dissolving form of lansoprazole and a powdered form of omeprazole are available for nasogastric tube administration.

Proton pump inhibitors are extensively metabolized by the CYP 450 enzymes, primarily CYP3A4 and CYP2C19.[14] CYP2C19 polymorphisms can significantly affect the metabolism of omeprazole and esomeprazole. Extensive metabolizers of omeprazole may require higher doses to achieve the same pharmacologic effect that poor metabolizers achieve on standard doses. Extensive metabolizers have been identified in 18% of the Swedish and Ethiopian populations but only 4% of the Chinese population. CYP2C19 activity has been shown to decline with age, such that even among extensive metabolizers, the metabolism of omeprazole is closer to that of poor metabolizers in much younger subjects.[15] The net effect of the variances in CYP2C19 genotype and age are likely to result in the need for standard omeprazole dosing in most patients. Those extensive metabolizers with normal or intact CYP2C19 activity may be candidates for high-dose omeprazole but dosage should be governed by clinical response to therapy. The other proton pump inhibitors are metabolized to a much lesser extent or not at all by CYP2C19 and therefore are less likely to be affected by either the rapid CYP2C19 genotype or the decline in CYP2C19 function with age.[14]

None of the proton pump inhibitors require dosage adjustment in patients with renal impairment, whereas the dosage of pantoprazole and rabeprazole should be decreased and these drugs should be used cautiously in patients with hepatic impairment.[11]

Histamine-2 Receptor Antagonists

Important differences exist among histamine-2 antagonists that should be considered when selecting one of these agents in older persons. Cimetidine can cause thrombocytopenia, neutropenia, bradycardia, arrhythmias, confusion, depression, and gynecomastia. Cimetidine is associated with more clinically important drug interactions than the other histamine-2 antagonists because it inhibits CYP3A4 and CYP2C19 enzymes thereby decreasing the metabolism and increasing the effect of warfarin, phenytoin, theophylline, and some benzodiazepines.[10,11] For these reasons and because of the larger frequency and severity of adverse reactions, cimetidine is not recommended in the elderly.[11] Cimetidine and ranitidine have been reported to cause dyskinesia, whereas famotidine and cimetidine can cause impotence, particularly in high doses.[10,11] Ranitidine has been found to have significant anticholinergic properties that may contribute to cognitive decline, constipation, dry eyes, and urinary retention in susceptible patients.[11,16] Headache occurs in 4.7% and 3% of patients treated with famotidine and ranitidine, respectively.[11] Ranitidine may inhibit CYP isozymes but famotidine and nizatidine are not metabolized by the CYP isoenzymes and do not have an inhibitory effect on hepatic clearance of other medications.[11] All histamine-2 antagonists can cause reversible central nervous system side effects and thrombocytopenia.

All of the histamine-2 antagonists are cleared by glomerular filtration and dose reduction, by extending the dosing interval, is recommended even in persons with mild to moderate decreases in CrCl (ie, 30–60 mL/min). With severe renal impairment (CrCl <30 mL/min) the dosing interval should be extended further, the dose decreased, and patients observed for adverse central nervous system side effects.[10,11]

Laxatives

All categories of laxatives can cause bloating, flatulence, and abdominal pain.[17] Bulk-forming laxatives (eg, psyllium, methylcellulose, and polycarbophil) can cause constipation or impaction if they are not taken with sufficient fluids.[17] Patients should be instructed to drink at least 250 mL of liquid with each dose of a bulk-forming laxative. As this level of fluid intake can be difficult for frail older persons with swallowing difficulties who drink inadequate volumes of fluid, bulk-forming laxatives may not be a good choice.

Osmotic laxatives are generally safe and effective in older persons but should not be used in patients with renal, liver, or heart failure.[17] Emollient laxatives, specifically mineral oil, can cause lipid pneumonitis in older patients if aspirated and will decrease absorption of fat-soluble vitamins if taken chronically. For these reasons, mineral oil is not recommended as a laxative in older persons.[17,18] Stool softeners, such as docusate are generally well tolerated in older persons. Saline laxatives have been associated with significant cramping, flatulence, and electrolyte disturbances. Long-term use of stimulant laxatives is not recommended as they become habit-forming, and have been associated with electrolyte disturbances.

Lubiprostone causes a dose-dependent nausea, which is offset somewhat by ingesting with food. Methylnaltrexone is generally well tolerated with abdominal pain, flatulence, nausea, dizziness, and diarrhea reported in greater than 5% of patients.[17]

Magnesium citrate and magnesium hydroxide (MOM) should be used with caution in patients with mild to moderate renal impairment, whereas sodium phosphate is contraindicated. In patients with severe renal impairment (CrCl <30 mL/min) sorbitol, magnesium citrate, and MOM are contraindicated.

Antiemetics

Older persons can have symptoms of nausea and vomiting caused by medications, cancer, other illnesses, and constipation. When known, the choice of antiemetic can be selected by the receptor associated with the potential cause. For example, prokinetic agents (ie, metoclopramide) can be prescribed for gastric stasis, a neuroleptic for drug-induced nausea, an antihistamine for motion sickness, and a benzodiazepine for anticipatory nausea. However, empiric drug selection can be equally effective as many older persons are unable to provide a cause or describe their symptomatology in specific terms.[19] Drug-related causes should be investigated and offending agents discontinued whenever possible.

Dopaminergic agents, like haloperidol, are effective for treating intractable nausea and vomiting and in opioid-associated nausea.[19] Phenothiazines, such as prochlorperazine or chlorperazine, are useful for patients with nausea as a result of intestinal obstruction. Anticholinergic agents for nausea that also decrease secretions include hyoscyamine or scopolamine. However, the greater the anticholinergic effects, the more likely the agent will produce unwanted side effects in older persons. Metoclopramide, which has anticholinergic and dopaminergic effects, also inhibits serotonin receptors at higher doses.

Serotonin receptor antagonists, ondansetron, granisetron, and dolasetron have well-defined roles in postoperative nausea and vomiting as well as radiation-induced nausea.[17] They can be used alone or combined with corticosteroids, such as dexamethasone for treating chemotherapy-induced nausea and vomiting. Corticosteroids can be effective in treating nausea related to bowel obstruction.[17] Because dexamethasone lacks mineralocorticoid properties, it is the preferred corticosteroid for older persons.

In older persons many antiemetic agents are associated with undesirable consequences. Benzodiazepines can impair cognitive function and have been associated with hip fracture.[20] Dosage reduction is recommended for older persons with hepatic impairment for all benzodiazepines except lorazepam, oxazepam, and temazepam, which undergo glucuronidation.[19] In older persons, metoclopramide is associated with dyskinesia, anxiety, depression, insomnia, hallucination, fatigue, drowsiness, tremor, and restlessness.[19] If metoclopramide is prescribed, The Abnormal Involuntary Movement Scale should be used for monitoring therapy.[19] Metoclopramide dosage reduction is recommended in persons with renal impairment (ClCr <40 mL/min).[10] Anticholinergic agents, like scopolamine or hyoscyamine, are associated with constipation, dry mouth, blurred vision, urinary retention, drowsiness, and tachycardia and are poor choices in older persons.[10]

Antidiarrheals

None-infectious diarrhea can be treated safely and effectively with bismuth subsalicylate or loperamide in older persons because of the favorable safety profile.[21] Loperamide should be avoided when there are features of mucosal involvement such as bleeding and if diarrhea induced by *C difficile* is suspected. Loperamide can cause central nervous system effects in patients with hepatic impairment and causes spasm of the sphincter of Oddi, thereby increasing serum amylase and lipase concentrations in some patients.[10] Antiperistaltic agents, such as diphenoxylate, can produce nausea, lightheadedness, confusion, and sedation, and should not be used in persons with infectious diarrhea.[21] Diphenoxylate is contraindicated in persons with jaundice or hepatic impairment. Bismuth subsalicylate is effective in the treatment of nonspecific causes of diarrhea. The salicylate component of bismuth subsalicylate can be absorbed in sufficient quantities to cause bleeding and should not be combined for more than a day or two with salicylate therapy without monitoring serum concentrations of salicylate. Opium and paregoric are considered unacceptable for use in older persons because of the potential for adverse central nervous system effects.[21]

Possible drug-related causes of diarrhea should be investigated and alternative medications selected whenever possible.

Antispasmodics

Antispasmodics are still in widespread use in nursing home residents despite cautions against their use.[18,22] "Antispasmodic drugs are poorly tolerated by elderly patients, since they cause anticholinergic adverse effects, sedation, and weakness. Additionally, their effectiveness at doses tolerated by older persons is questionable."[18] For these reasons belladonna alkaloids, hyoscyamine, dicyclomine, and propantheline are considered unacceptable for use in older persons.

Benzodiazepines are used as antispasmodics in persons with GI cramping, nausea, and diarrhea. However, long-acting benzodiazepines, such as chlordiazepoxide have been associated with hip fracture and because they accumulate even in short-term use, contribute to confusion and cognitive decline in susceptible patients.[20] There are no safe alternatives to these medications in older persons.

PREVENTABLE DRUG-INDUCED GI CONDITIONS

Drug-related conditions have been estimated to account for $138 to $182 billion in total cost in 1994 when the estimated cost of drug-related adverse effects exceeded the cost of drugs in the United States and became the fifth most expensive condition.[23] Drug-induced GI conditions can include nausea and vomiting, constipation, infectious and noninfectious diarrhea, liver disease, upper GI bleeding, gastric erosions, and gastroesophageal reflux disease (GERD). In a retrospective cohort study of adverse drug reactions in persons older than 60 years of age, nausea and vomiting (8%) were the most common adverse events accounting for repeat hospital admission.[24] Gurwitz and colleagues[25] identified GI tract events (eg, nausea, vomiting, diarrhea, constipation, and abdominal pain) as the most common type of preventable adverse drug event (22.1%) in their analysis of adverse drug events in older ambulatory persons. The list of medications associated with drug-induced nausea, vomiting, diarrhea, constipation, and abdominal pain is extensive.[10] **Table 2** summarizes a few preventable drug-induced GI conditions that are widely reported in older persons.

Drug-Induced Diarrhea

Drugs can induce osmotic, secretory, or inflammatory diarrhea, diarrhea caused from disordered motility, or infectious diarrhea (pseudomembranous colitis).[26] More than 700 medications have been implicated in causing diarrhea but in some cases the mechanism of action is not clear. When diarrhea is watery, it can be either osmotic or secretory. Osmotic diarrhea is caused by medications such as magnesium-containing salts and laxatives, such as polyethylene glycol. These products draw water into the GI tract. Acarbose and miglitol used for the treatment of type 2 diabetes prevent the breakdown of carbohydrates to monosaccharides by inhibiting intestinal a-glucosidase and result in diarrhea in as many as 30% of patients. Secretory diarrhea occurs when sodium ion absorption is impaired and chloride and bicarbonate ions are secreted into the lumen of the GI tract.[26] Absorption of water is impaired and secretory diarrhea results. A large number of medications commonly used in the elderly can induce secretory diarrhea including antibiotics, anticholinergics, metformin, digoxin, carbamazepine, cholinesterase inhibitors, cimetidine, anti-inflammatory drugs (NSAIDs), olsalazine, simvastatin, stimulant laxatives, theophylline, and ticlopidine.[26] Disordered motility can result from medications that alter the cholinergic system or cause prokinesis (eg, metoclopramide and erythromycin). Bethanechol, cholinesterase inhibitors, metoclopramide, erythromycin, and excess levothyroxine are commonly associated with diarrhea resulting from disordered motility.

Inflammatory diarrhea is described as disruption of colonic flora precipitating C difficile colitis, or following direct damage of the gastric mucosa.[26] Many antibiotics have been associated with causing C difficile diarrhea (**Table 2**).[27] Even brief exposure to antibiotics can result in C difficile colitis, but a prolonged course of treatment or prescription of two or more antibiotics increases the risk as does increasing age, severity of underlying disease, presence of a nasogastric tube, acid reduction therapy, recent or prolonged hospitalization, and repeated antibiotic treatments.[28,29] Nonantibiotic causes of C difficile diarrhea are proton pump inhibitors, histamine-2 receptor antagonists, and immunosuppressants as a result of disruption of the acid-base environment or epithelial homeostasis. The result is superficial necrosis and an imbalance of secretory, absorptive, and motility functions of the gut, contributing to diarrhea.[26]

NSAIDs cause diarrhea in 3% to 9% of patients by stimulating in vitro absorption of sodium ions but also through increased permeability and direct mucosal damage. In addition, NSAIDs have been associated with pseudomembranous colitis.[26]

Fatty diarrhea occurs if there is maldigestion or malabsorption of fat. Several HIV medications produce steatorrhea; antiretrovirals, nucleoside analog reverse transcriptase inhibitors (17%–28%) and protease inhibitors (52%) cause diarrhea.[26] orlistat, a weight loss drug, and alli (a derivative of orlistat) cause steatorrhea in as many as

Table 2
Drug-induced GI conditions

C difficile Diarrhea	
Frequently associated	Ampicillin, amoxicillin and derivatives, first, second and third generation cephalosporins, imipenem/cilastatin, clindamycin
Occasionally associated	Ertapenem, meropenem, ciprofloxacin, gatifloxacin, levofloxacin, moxifloxacin, norflaxacin, azithromycin, clarithromycin, erythromycin, pencillicins, carbenicillin, dicloxacillin, mezlocillin, nafcillin, oxacillin, piperacillin, ticarcillin, sulfonamides, proton pump inhibitors
Less commonly associated	Amikacin, gentamicin, kanamycin, neomycin, streptomycin, tobramycin, vancomycin, aztreonam, dalfopristin/quinupristin, fosfomycin, linezolid, loracarbef, metronidazole, nitrofurantoin, rifampin, doxycycline, minocycline, tetracycline
Noninfectious diarrhea	
Watery diarrhea	α-Glucosidase inhibitors: acarbose, miglitol
Secretory diarrhea	Antibiotics, anticholinergics, auranofin, metformin, digoxin, calcitonin, carbamazepine, cholinesterase inhibitors, cimetidine, NSAIDs, simvastatin, theophylline
Altered motility	Cholinergic drugs, macrolide antibiotics, metoclopramide
Inflammatory diarrhea	Antibiotics, carbamazepine, chemotherapeutic agents (5-fluorouracil, cisplatin, irinotecan), immunosuppressive agents (methotrexate, mycophenol, mofetil), NSAIDs, proton pump inhibitors, SSRIs (sertraline), tyrosine kinase inhibitors (erlotinib, gefitinib, imatinib)
Fatty diarrhea	Metformin, HIV medications, octreotide, orlistat, cholestyramine, tetracyclines
Constipation	
More commonly associated	Antacids: aluminum- and calcium-containing
	Anticonvulsants: lacosamide, carbamazepine, phenytoin
	Anticholinergic agents (**Table 3**)
	Antipsychotics: quetiapine, risperidone, aripiprazole, clozapine
	Ferrous salts
	Dopamine agonists: pramipexole, ropinirole
	Tricyclic antidepressants
	Calcium channel blockers: verapamil, diltiazem
Less commonly associated	Anticonvulsants: lamotrigine, valproic acid
	Antipsychotics: olanzapine
	Calcium channel blockers: dihydropyridine, amlodipine

Bleeding, erosions, GERD, NERD	Aspirin, NSAIDs, COX-2s Potassium salts Anti-infectives: amoxicillin, ciprofloxacin, clindamycin, TMP/SMX, erythromycin, tetracyclines Bisphosphonates: alendronate, etidronate, ibandronate, risedronate, tiludronate Ferrous salts Memantine Quinidine Theophylline
Pill esophagitis	Potassium salts: SR tablets SR products, especially solid oral tablets and osmotic drug release technology Bisphosphonates Tetracyclines NSAIDs
Liver toxicity	
Cholestatic injury, ALK>2>ULN, ALT:ALK ratio <2	Anabolic and contraceptive steroids Phenothiazine antipsychotics: proclorperazine, chlorpromazine Antibiotics: erythromycins, amoxicillin-clavulanate, sulfonamides (TMP/SMX), nitrofurantoin Carbamazepine Cyclosporine NSAIDS: sulindac, naproxen ACEIs, ARBs
Cytotoxic/hepatocellular injury, ALT>2×ULN, ALT:ALK ratio >5	Analgesics: acetaminophen, aspirin, diclofenac, indomethacin, ketorolac, ibuprofen, ketoprofen Anti-infectives: isoniazid, itraconazole, ketoconazole, liposomal amphotericin B, nitrofurantoin, sulfonamides Ferrous salts Antihypertensives: methydopa, hydralazine, labetolol Anticonvulsants: carbamazepine, valproic acid

Abbreviations: ACEIs, angiotensin converting enzyme inhibitors; ALK, alanine phosphatase; ALT, alanine aminotransferase; ARBs, angiotensin receptor blockers; COX-2s, cyclooxygenase-2 selective inhibitors; GERD, gastroesophageal reflux disease; NERD, nonerosive reflux disease; NSAIDs, nonsteroidal anti-inflammatory drugs; SR, sustained-release; SSRIs, selective serotonin reuptake inhibitors; TMP/SMX, trimethoprim/sulfamethoxazole; ULN, upper limit of normal.
Data from Refs.[10,13,16,17,21,26,27,30–32,38–41,44–46]

60% to 80% of patients. In high doses (24–30 g/d), cholestyramine can cause steatorrhea.[26] Metformin can cause a malabsorptive diarrhea as a result of reduction of disaccharidase activity.[10] Paradoxically, at higher doses octreotide can actually cause fatty diarrhea despite being indicated as an antidiarrheal agent.[26]

Strategies to avoid drug-induced diarrhea vary with the causative agent and may include avoidance of unnecessary drug treatment (ie, antibiotics for viral infection), selection of an alternative agent in the same class or a different drug class (ie, insulin instead of metformin or acarbose for type 2 diabetes), slow initiation and titration of drug therapy, and use of concomitant antidiarrheals such as diphenoxylate, loperamide, or bismuth subsalicylate. Treatment of drug-induced diarrhea usually involves removal or reduction in dosage of the offending agent and may require the addition of specific medications such as metronidazole or oral vancomycin for treatment of *C difficile* diarrhea.[27]

Constipation

Constipation can be induced by medications with anticholinergic potential (**Table 3**) and others that slow transit through the colon. Dopamine agonists, tricylic antidepressants, antipsychotics medications, calcium channel blockers, opioid analgesics, and calcium/aluminum-containing antacids have been implicated in causing or worsening constipation in older persons. Underlying conditions contribute to slow transit, which is exaggerated by low fiber intake and anticholinergic medications.[30] Disordered defecation of aging and underlying conditions can contribute to fecal incontinence and fecal impaction. Assessment and management of constipation in older persons is addressed elsewhere in this issue.

Gastric Mucosal Damage, Bleeding, and Ulceration

In addition to an association with drug-induced diarrhea, NSAIDs, including cyclooxygenase-2 selective inhibitors (COX-2), and aspirin are implicated in causing GI hemorrhage, stricture, and ulceration.[31] NSAIDs can cause damage throughout the GI tract, but the predominant site of injury is the stomach. Dyspepsia is common with NSAIDs and equally common with COX-2 selective and nonselective drugs. Serious upper GI events such as perforation and bleeding from gastric or duodenal ulcers occur in up to 2% of NSAID users. Bleeding and perforation are often not heralded by symptoms. Endoscopic lesions are a poor surrogate for upper GI bleeding or perforation.[32] NSAIDs cause local effects such as hyperemia, erosions, and subepithelial hemorrhages and systemic effects secondary to prostaglandin inhibition.[31] Prostaglandins are cytoprotective to the gastric mucosa by maintaining blood flow, increasing secretion of mucus and bicarbonate and by augmenting epithelial defense against cytotoxic injury. When prostaglandins are inhibited by NSAIDs, aspirin, or less selective COX-2 agents, ulceration of the gastric mucosa can occur. Symptomatic ulcers and ulcer complications, such as bleeding and perforation are serious, potentially life-threatening consequences of NSAID therapy.[31]

Strategies to reduce the risk of gastric mucosa damage involve avoiding the use of NSAIDs, aspirin, and COX-2 agents in elderly persons who have been characterized to be at high risk for GI damage and bleeding. When these agents are necessary, use of a more COX-2 selective medication, such as celecoxib or meloxicam reduces the number of GI-related adverse events and related withdrawals when compared with nonselective NSAIDs.[32] Following analysis of published trials, the Health Technology Assessment (HTA) report concluded that meloxicam reduces the relative risk (RR) of clinical GI events (RR 0.42, 95% CI 0.26–0.72) and complicated upper GI events (RR 0.44, 95% CI 0.23–0.85) compared with nonselective NSAIDS.[32] Celecoxib was

Table 3
Alternative medications with lower anticholinergic burden

Drug Class	High Anticholinergic Potential	Alternatives with Lower Anticholinergic Potential
Anxiolytics and sedative hypnotics	Chlordiazepoxide Diazepam Flurazepam Temazepam	Alprazolam Lorazepam Oxazepam Zaleplon Zolpidem
Corticosteroids	Dexamethasone Hydrocortisone Prednisolone	
Antidepressants	Amitriptyline Doxepin Nortriptyline Paroxetine	Bupropion Sertraline Trazodone Venlafaxine Duloxetine
Antihistamines	Diphenhydramine	Cetirizine Fexofenadine Loratadine
Antipsychotics	Clozapine Thioridazine Chlorpromazine Olanzapine Quetiapine	Aripiprazole Haloperidol Perphenazine Risperidone Ziprasidone
Antispasmodics	Belladonna Clidinium-chlordiazepoxide Dicyclomine Hyoscyamine Propantheline	
Antidiarrheals	Diphenoxylate	Bisacodyl
Antinauseants	Metoclopramide Phenothiazines	5-HT$_3$ antagonists: dolasetron, ondansetron, granisetron
Histamine-2 receptor antagonists	Ranitidine	Famotidine or a proton pump inhibitor
Mood stabilizers	Lithium	Carbamazepine Gabapentin Lamotrigine Valproate
Muscle relaxants	Carisoprodol Chlorzoxazone Cyclobenzaprine Metaxalone Methocarbamol	Baclofen

Abbreviation: 5-HT$_3$, 5-hydroxytryptamine 3 receptor.
Data from Refs.[16,47,48]

associated with significantly fewer GI withdrawals, fewer endoscopic GI ulcers and significantly fewer clinical (RR 0.55, 95% CI 0.4–0.76) and complicated upper GI events (RR 0.57, 95% CI 0.35–0.95) compared with nonselective NSAIDs. Meloxicam seems to reduce the risk of upper GI events and complications better than nonselective NSAIDs but not quite as effectively as celecoxib. However, HTA concluded an almost twofold increase in the RR of myocardial infarction (MI) with celecoxib compared with nonselective NSAIDs (RR 1.72, 95% CI 1.00–3.11).[32] The increased risk appeared to be independent of celecoxib dose. It seems that the benefit of reduced GI damage and significant clinical events may be offset somewhat by an increased risk of cardiovascular events as COX-2 selectivity increases. The highest associated rates of MI and stroke occur with the most highly COX-2 selective NSAIDs.[33]

A second strategy to reduce GI damage if NSAIDs and COX-2s are necessary, is the addition of a prostaglandin analog, such as misoprostol, or suppression of gastric acid production with a proton pump inhibitor. Because of the high occurrence of diarrhea with misoprostol and the effectiveness and safety of proton pump inhibitors, the recent statement from the American College of Cardiology and the American College of Gastroenterology recommends the addition of a proton pump inhibitor to all NSAID therapy in high-risk patients (>65 years) irrespective of COX-2 selectively.[34] Proton pump inhibitors are associated with superior effectiveness and safety compared with histamine-2 receptor antagonists and are recommended as first line protective therapy when NSAIDs are prescribed.[35] Histamine-2 receptor antagonists protect against duodenal but not gastric ulceration, whereas proton pump inhibitors protect against gastric and duodenal erosion. Although low-dose aspirin may be a less well-recognized cause of gastric ulceration, doses as low as 10 mg/d can be ulceragenic.[36]

Iron is directly corrosive to the gastric mucosa and can cause ischemic lesions, necrosis, and ulceration.[31] For these reasons and limitations in iron absorption, the dose of iron is typically limited to no more than 325 mg/d of ferrous sulfate or equivalent of other available salts.[18]

Older persons who have received erosive or corrosive drug therapy who present with symptoms of upper GI bleeding or ulceration (alarm symptoms), should be evaluated for *Helicobacter pylori* as it is easily treatable if present. The American College of Gastroenterology recommends ruling out cancer in persons older than 55 years of age before treatment remedies are undertaken.[37]

Pill Esophagitis

Older persons, particularly residents of long-term care facilities, exhibit risk factors for the development of pill-induced esophagitis and dysphagia including old age, institutionalization, preexisting esophageal or swallowing disorders, recumbent position, prescription of gelatin capsules, and extended- or sustained-release products.[38] Conditions prevalent in older persons can alter GI transit and predispose affected patients to an increased risk of pill-induced esophagitis, such as Parkinsons disease, neurologic impairment, cerebrovascular accidents, myasthenia gravis, preexisting stricture, reflux disease, or hiatal hernia. In residents of long-term care facilities, the use of conventional antipsychotic agents further increases the risk of pill-induced esophagitis secondary to the antidopaminergic activity, particularly of higher potency agents. Atypical antipsychotics are preferred when treatment with a neuroleptic is needed because of the lower incidence of drug-induced Parkinsonism and tardive dyskinesia and decreased risk of swallowing dysfunction.[38] Drug-induced esophageal injury has been described with many medications including tetracyclines, bisphosphonates (eg, alendronate risedronate), nonsteroidal anti-inflammatory drugs, and quinidine.[38,39] Long-acting, enteric-coated and slow-release oral solids designed to provide more consistent serum concentrations are more likely to be associated with pill-induced esophagitis than immediate-release or liquid preparations.[38] Drug-induced esophagitis presents with a feeling that the pill is stuck in the throat. Patients may complain of burning and retrosternal pain. Drug-induced damage usually heals in a few days without sequelae, but if unresolved and left untreated, has been associated with malnutrition, esophageal perforation, hemorrhage, and death.

There are reports in the literature of enteric-coated potassium chloride formulations causing severe esophageal damage and death.[38–42] Extended-release and wax matrix tablets are implicated more often than liquid or powder formulations (**Table 2**).[38] Older persons are predisposed to drug-induced esophageal damage as a result of declining motility and saliva production with age.[43]

The risk of pill-induced esophagitis can be decreased in susceptible patients by administering medications only in the upright position, followed by a full glass of water and avoiding sustained-release tablet formulations of potassium chloride. Whenever possible, medications with anticholinergic potential should be avoided in older adults. Not only do anticholinergics predispose older patients to confusion, urinary retention, and cardiac consequences, but because of the delay in gastric emptying and drying of oral and gastric secretions, anticholinergics predispose individuals to pill-induced esophagitis.

Liver Toxicity

More than 800 medications have been associated with hepatotoxicty.[44] Drug-induced liver disease accounts for 2% to 16% of hospital admissions. Medicines account for approximately 50% of the cases of liver failure that occur annually in the United States. Patterns of drug-induced hepatic disease include cytotoxic, cholestatic, vascular, and neoplastic injury. Risk factors for increased susceptibility to drug-induced liver disease are female gender (nitrofurantoin, sulfonamides), male gender (azathioprine, amoxicillin-clavulanate), older than 65 years of age (isoniazid, amoxicillin-clavulanate), and malnutrition or fasting (acetaminophen).[45] In older persons, commonly used medications that pose the greatest risk of hepatoxicity are acetaminophen, phenytoin, carbamazepine, valproic acid, vitamin A, ferrous salts, and methotrexate.[45] **Table 2** provides examples of each major type of liver toxicity.

Frail older persons may be at increased risk of acetaminophen-induced liver toxicity.[45] Frail older persons who are malnourished may have inadequate stores of glutathione in the liver. Glutathione conjugates acetaminophen's toxic metabolite (N-acetyl-p-benzoquinone imine) to a nontoxic metabolite, which is then eliminated renally. Acetaminophen-induced hepatoxicity can occur at lower doses in older persons because production of N-acetyl-p-benzoquinone imine increases with age greater than 65 years.[45,46] For these reasons, it may be reasonable to limit total daily doses of acetaminophen in older cachectic persons to less than the conventionally recommended 4 g/d, although no specific recommendations exist.

Management of patients at risk of drug-induced liver toxicity involves identification and discontinuation of the offending agent. Symptoms of liver toxicity, such as hepatitis, and elevated liver transaminases generally return to normal in 2 to 3 weeks following drug discontinuation. Specific strategies do not exist for most medications and care is generally supportive. N-Acetylcysteine is a specific antidote for acetaminophen toxicity whether by acute or chronic ingestion. N-Acetylcysteine replenishes glutathione stores and causes vasodilation, which increases tissue oxygen uptake. It has antioxidant properties and suppresses tumor necrosis factor.[46]

GI Drugs to Avoid in the Elderly

Despite the effectiveness of selected medications in older persons with GI disorders, there are substantial differences in comparative safety or potential for adverse events among agents. In most drug classes used to treat GI conditions there is at least one choice with a lower potential to cause drug-related adverse events.

Medications with anticholinergic properties pose risks of constipation, urinary retention, dry eyes, confusion, dizziness, and falls. Medications that antagonize muscarinic receptor activity can impair cognitive functions such as working memory, episodic memory, processing speed, and praxis.[16] The anticholinergic burden of numerous medications has been characterized, which can guide clinicians in the choice of safer medications.[16,47] Through the in vitro application of a radioreceptor assay, investigators quantified the anticholinergic activity of 107 medications at various therapeutic concentrations that result when these agents are prescribed.[16] Although this model did not account for the differences in penetration into the central nervous system, the study findings can be helpful to guide clinicians on the selection of medications with lower anticholinergic potential in older patients. **Table 3** summarizes GI drugs with high anticholinergic potential and suggested alternatives with lower anticholinergic burden.[16,48]

SUMMARY

The effects of medications on the GI tract and related organs can significantly alter the expected therapeutic result and contribute to adverse outcomes. Because of the natural consequences of aging superimposed on progression of chronic underlying conditions, the elderly are more likely to be subject to changes in drug effects and adverse events. Clinicians are challenged to avoid selection of medications that are likely to induce adverse GI consequences, and those subject to therapeutic failure in older persons.

Reconciliation of medication lists, use of interdisciplinary teams, clinical algorithms, care plans or clinical pathways, and the application of health information technology are strategies employed in many acute care institutions and long-term facilities to improve medication safety in vulnerable elders. The continued expansion of geriatric training in undergraduate, graduate, and postgraduate education is needed to adequately prepare health care professionals for the challenges they face in managing drug therapy in the frail elderly. The tenet of "start low" and "go slow" does not adequately account for the complex pharmacokinetic and pharmacodynamic implications of drug therapy in the aging. Unless the use of a given medication, at the dose selected, is determined to have benefited the patient, further evaluation with either adjustment in dosage or discontinuation should be considered.

REFERENCES

1. Relay health claims data warehouse. Atlanta (GA): Omnicare, Inc.; 2008.
2. Elliott DP. Pharmacokinetics and pharmacodynamics in the elderly. In: Schumock GI, Brundage DM, Hammond Chessman K, et al, editors. Pharmacotherapy self-assessment program, 5th edition. Geriatrics and special populations book of PSAP-V. Kansas City (MO): American College of Clinical Pharmacy; 2005. p. 115–26.
3. McLean AJ, Le Couteur DG. Aging biology and geriatric clinical pharmacology. Pharmacol Rev 2004;56:163–84.
4. Lindeman RD, Tobin J, Shock NW. Longitudinal studies on the rate of decline in renal function with age. J Am Geriatr Soc 1985;33:278–85.
5. Giannelli SV, Patel KV, Windham BG, et al. Magnitude of underascertainment of impaired kidney function in older adults with normal serum creatinine. J Am Geriatr Soc 2007;816–23.
6. Levey AS, Bosch JP, Lewis JB, et al. A more accurate method to estimate glomerular filtration rate from serum creatinine: a new prediction equation. Modification of Diet in Renal Disease Study Group. Ann Intern Med 1999;130:461–70.

7. Cockcroft DW, Gault MH. Prediction of creatinine clearance from serum creatinine. Nephron 1976;16:31–41.
8. K/DOQI Clinical practice guidelines for chronic kidney disease: evaluation, classification, and stratification. Kidney disease outcome quality initiative. Am J Kidney Dis 2002;39:S1–246.
9. Hanlon JT, Aspinall SL, Semla TP, et al. Consensus guidelines for oral dosing of primarily renally cleared medications in older adults. J Am Geriatr Soc 2008; EOI:10.1111/j.1532–5415.2008.0298.x.
10. Clinical Pharmacology Online. Gold Standard, an Elsevier Company: Tampa (FL); 2009. Available at: http://www.clinicalpharmacology.com/accessed. Accessed March 21, 2009.
11. Gastroesophageal reflux disease. In: Geriatric pharmaceutical care guidelines. Covington (KY): Omnicare, Inc.; 2009. p. 423–9.
12. Yang YX, Lewis JD, Epstein S, et al. Long-term proton pump inhibitor use and the risk of hip fracture. JAMA 2006;296:2947–53.
13. Dial S, Delaney JA, Barkun AN, et al. Use of gastric acid-suppressive agents and the risk of community-acquired Clostridium difficile-associated disease. JAMA 2005;294:2989–95.
14. Shi S, Klotz U. Proton pump inhibitors: an update of their clinical use and pharmacokinetics. Eur J Clin Pharmacol 2008;64:935–51.
15. Ishizawa Y, Yasui-Furukori N, Takahata T, et al. The effect of aging on the relationship between the cytochrome P450 2C19 genotype and omeprazole pharmacokinetics. Clin Pharmacokinet 2005;44:1179–89.
16. Chew M, Mulsant BH, Pollock BG, et al. Anticholinergic activity of 107 medications commonly used by older adults. J Am Geriatr Soc 2008;56:1333–41.
17. Constipation. In: Geriatric pharmaceutical care guidelines. Covington (KY): Omnicare, Inc.; 2009. p. 257–68.
18. Fick DM, Cooper JW, Wade WE, et al. Updating the Beers criteria for potentially inappropriate medication use in older adults. Arch Intern Med 2003;163:2716–24.
19. Palliative care, pharmacotherapy. In: Geriatric pharmaceutical care guidelines. Covington (KY): Omnicare, Inc.; 2009. p. 661–75.
20. Wagner AK, Zhang F, Soumerai SB, et al. Benzodiazepine use and hip fractures in the elderly: who is at greatest risk? Arch Intern Med 2004;164:1567–72.
21. Diarrhea: noninfectious. In: Geriatric pharmaceutical care guidelines. Covington (KY): Omnicare, Inc.; 2009. p. 387–93.
22. Curtis LH, Østbye T, Sendersky V, et al. Inappropriate prescribing for elderly American in a large outpatient population. Arch Intern Med 2004;164:1621–5.
23. Johnson JA, Bootman LJ. Drug-related morbidity and mortality: a cost-of-illness model. Arch Intern Med 1995;155:1949–56.
24. Zhang M, Holman DJ, Preen DB. Repeat adverse drug reactions causing hospitalization in older Australians: a population-based longitudinal study 1980–2003. Br J Clin Pharmacol 2006;63:163–70.
25. Gurwitz JH, Field TS, Harrold LR, et al. Incidence and preventability of adverse drug events among older persons in the ambulatory setting. JAMA 2003;289:1107–16.
26. Abraham B, Sellin JH. Drug-induced diarrhea. Curr Gastroenterol Rep 2007;9:365–72.
27. Diarrhea: Clostridium difficile-associated. Geriatric pharmaceutical care guidelines. Covington (KY): Omnicare, Inc.; 2009. p. 373–85.
28. Owens RC. Clostridium difficile-associated disease: an emerging threat to patient safety. Pharmacother 2006;26:299–311.

29. Bartlett JG. Narrative review: the new epidemic of *Clostridium difficile*-associated enteric disease. Ann Intern Med 2006;145:758–64.
30. Muller-Lissner S. General geriatrics and gastroenterology: constipation and faecal incontinence. Best Pract Res Clin Gastroenterol 2002;16:115–33.
31. Puszlaszeri MP, Genta RM, Cryer BL. Drug-induced injury in the gastrointestinal tract: clinical and pathologic considerations. Nat Clin Pract Gastroenterol Hepatol 2007;4(8):442–54.
32. Chen YF, Jobanputra P, Barton P, et al. Cyclooxygenase-2 selective non-steroidal anti-inflammatory drugs (etodolac, meloxicam, celecoxib, rofecoxib, etoricoxib, valdecoxib and lumiracoxib) for osteoarthritis and rheumatoid arthritis: a systematic review and economic evaluation. Health Technol Assess 2008;12:1–198. Available at: www.hta.ac.uk. Accessed March 21, 2009.
33. Abraham NS, El-Serag HB, Hartman C, et al. Cyclooxygenase-2 selectivity of non-steroidal anti-inflammatory drugs and the risk of myocardial infarction and cerebrovascular accident. Aliment Pharmacol Ther 2007;25:913–24.
34. Bhatt DL, Scheiman J, Abraham NS, et al. ACCF/ACG/AHA 2008 expert consensus document on reducing the gastrointestinal risks of antiplatelet therapy and NSAID use: a report of the American College of Cardiology Foundation Task Force on Clinical Expert Consensus Documents. Circulation 2008;118:1894–909.
35. Talley NJ. American gastroenterological association medical position statement: evaluation of dyspepsia. Gastroenterol 2005;129:1753–5.
36. Sapoznikov B, Vilkin A, Hershkovici M, et al. Minidose aspirin and gastrointestinal bleeding – a retrospective, case-control study in hospitalized patients. Dig Dis Sci 2005;50:1621–4.
37. Talley NJ, Vakil NB, Moayyedi P. American gastroenterological association technological review on the evaluation of dyspepsia. Gastroenterol 2005;129:1756–80.
38. O'Neill JL, Remington TL. Drug-induced esophageal injuries and dysphagia. Ann Pharmacother 2003;37:1675–84.
39. Jaspersen D. Drug-induced oesophageal disorders: pathogenesis incidence, prevention and management. Drug Saf 2000;22:237–49.
40. Sherman A, Bini EJ. Pill-induced gastric injury. Am J Gastroenterol 1999;94:511–3.
41. Kikendall JW, Friedman AC, Oyewole MA, et al. Pill-induced esophageal injury: case reports and review of the medical literature. Dig Dis Sci 1983;28:174–82.
42. Baley RT Jr, Bonavina L, McChesney L, et al. Factors influencing the transit of a gelatin capsule in the esophagus. Drug Intell Clin Pharm 1987;21:282–5.
43. Gastrointestinal disorders: aging and the gastrointestinal tract. In: Beers MH, Berkow R, editors. The Merck manual of geriatrics. 3rd edition. Whitehouse Station (NJ): Merck Research Laboratories; 2000. p. 1000–42.
44. McLaren R. Drug-induced liver disease. In: Mueller BA, Bertch KE, Dunsworth TS, et al, editors. Pharmacotherapy self-assessment program, 4th edition. Gastroenterology, nutrition – PSAP-IV. Kansas City (MO): American College of Clinical Pharmacy; 2002. p. 139–58.
45. Kim J. Drug-induced liver disease. In: Richardson M, Chant C, Cheng JWM, Chessman KH, Hume AL, Hutchison LC, et al, editors. Pharmacotherapy Self-Assessment Program, 6th edition. Gastroenterology and nutrition – PSAP-VI. Lenexa (KS): American College of Clinical Pharmacy; 2009. p. 25–40.
46. Larson AM. Acetaminophen hepatotoxicity. Clin Liver Dis 2007;11:525–48.
47. Tune LE. Anticholinergic effects of medication in elderly patients. J Clin Psychiatry 2001;62(Suppl 21):11–4.
48. Medications with the potential for significant anticholinergic symptoms. Geriatric pharmaceutical care guidelines. Covington (KY): Omnicare, Inc.; 2009. p. 1033–34.

Index

Note: Page numbers of article titles are in **boldface** type.

A

Abscess, in diverticulitis, 515, 518
Absorption, drug, 547–548
Acetaminophen, hepatotoxicity of, 559
Adalimumab, for inflammatory bowel disease, 451
Addison disease, diarrhea in, 486
Adipose tissue, distribution of, 396–397, 399
Adrenal insufficiency, diarrhea in, 486
Allopurinol, for inflammatory bowel disease, 451
Anal manometry, in constipation, 471
Anal sphincter repair, for incontinence, 505
Analgesia, for diverticulitis, 518
Androgen deficiency, anorexia in, 403–404
Anemia, in celiac disease, 435
Angiography, in intestinal ischemia, 530–531, 535–536
Anorexia
    homeostasis impairment in, 397
    physiology of, 399–404
Antibiotics
    for diverticulitis, 518
    for intestinal ischemia, 532–533
    for small intestinal bacterial overgrowth, 491–492
Anticholinergic effects, of drugs, 556–557
Antidiarrheals, pharmacology of, 552
Antiemetics, pharmacology of, 551–552
Antiendomysial antibodies, in celiac disease, 437–438
Antispasmodics, pharmacology of, 552
Appetite loss, 399–400
Arterial embolism and thrombosis, in mesenteric ischemia, 529, 532–533
Aspiration, in dysphagia, 421
Aspirin, gastric damage due to, 555–558
Ataxia, in celiac disease, 439
Atherosclerosis, mesenteric ischemia in, 534
Autoimmune disorders, in celiac disease, 438–439
Azathioprine, for inflammatory bowel disease, 451

B

Bacterial overgrowth, small intestinal, 491–492
Baltimore Longitudinal Study of Aging, on drug elimination, 548

Gastroenterol Clin N Am 38 (2009) 563–575
doi:10.1016/S0889-8553(09)00084-3
0889-8553/09/$ – see front matter © 2009 Elsevier Inc. All rights reserved.

gastro.theclinics.com

Moving?

Make sure your subscription moves with you!

To notify us of your new address, find your **Clinics Account Number** (located on your mailing label above your name), and contact customer service at:

Email: journalscustomerservice-usa@elsevier.com

800-654-2452 (subscribers in the U.S. & Canada)
314-447-8871 (subscribers outside of the U.S. & Canada)

Fax number: 314-447-8029

Elsevier Health Sciences Division
Subscription Customer Service
3251 Riverport Lane
Maryland Heights, MO 63043

ELSEVIER

Printed and bound by CPI Group (UK) Ltd, Croydon, CR0 4YY

03/10/2024

01040464-0017